PLANT BASED DIET COOKBOOK FOR BEGINNERS 2024

Nourish Yourself with Some of the Best Plant-based Recipes.

FRANCIS A. CARTER

TABLE OF CONTENTS

Introduction

Dear Reader,

Welcome to a journey that promises not just delightful flavors, but a profound transformation of your relationship with food. In these pages lies a treasury of culinary discoveries that will guide you through the wondrous realm of a plant-based diet.

The decision to explore plant-based eating isn't just about what you place on your plate; it's a step toward nourishing your body, mind, and the environment. As the world evolves and our understanding of nutrition deepens, this cookbook aims to be your trusted companion, offering a gateway to a lifestyle that embraces health, sustainability, and culinary artistry.

In the chapters ahead, you'll find more than just recipes; you'll encounter a wealth of knowledge designed specifically for beginners. Whether you're taking your first steps into the world of plant-based eating or seeking inspiration to revitalize your meals, this book endeavors to be your steadfast guide.

Chapter 1: Understanding the Plant-Based Diet delves into the core principles, unraveling the science behind this lifestyle. It clarifies misconceptions and offers insights into the benefits, empowering you with the knowledge needed to embark on this journey confidently.

From sun-kissed mornings to comforting evenings, Chapters 2 to 4 introduce a plethora of recipes that will redefine your meals. Breakfasts that awaken your senses, Lunches that fuel your day, and Dinners that transform the ordinary into the extraordinary—all crafted with innovation and flavor in mind.

But the joy of dining isn't confined to main meals alone. Chapters 5 and 6 beckon you to explore the world of Appetizers that tease the palate and Treats that indulge your sweet cravings, proving that plant-based eating is anything but monotonous or limiting.

As you journey through these pages, savor the amalgamation of taste, health, and creativity. Each recipe, a testament to the infinite possibilities that plant-based ingredients offer, is a celebration of culinary diversity and nourishment.

And finally, in the Conclusion, take a moment to reflect on your newfound culinary voyage. Embrace the lessons learned, the flavors savored, and the transformations experienced.

Thank you for choosing to embark on this flavorful expedition with me. May these recipes not only tantalize your taste buds but also inspire a deeper connection with the food you consume and the world it stems from.

Bon appétit and happy cooking!

Warmest regards,

Francis A. Carter

Chapter 1

Understanding the Plant-Based Diet

A plant-based diet, at its core, revolves around the consumption of foods derived primarily from plants. This dietary approach emphasizes whole, minimally processed plant foods while minimizing or excluding animal products. It's often chosen for health, environmental, ethical, and religious reasons. The principles of a plant-based diet encompass various aspects, including its definition, types, health benefits, potential concerns, and practical tips for implementation.

Definition of a Plant-Based Diet

A plant-based diet is centered on plant-derived foods like vegetables, fruits, grains, legumes, nuts, seeds, and oils. The focus is on whole, nutrient-dense foods rather than heavily processed items. The diet encourages the intake of a wide variety of plant foods to ensure a diverse nutrient profile, including vitamins, minerals, fiber, and antioxidants.

Principles of a Plant-Based Diet

- Emphasis on Whole Foods: The diet prioritizes whole, unrefined foods, such as whole grains instead of refined grains, and encourages minimal processing to retain nutrients.

- Abundance of Fruits and Vegetables: These are rich sources of vitamins, minerals, antioxidants, and fiber. They constitute a significant portion of the diet.

- Inclusion of Legumes: Beans, lentils, and peas are staples in a plant-based diet, providing protein, fiber, and various essential nutrients.

- Grains and Tubers: Whole grains like quinoa, brown rice, and tubers like potatoes offer energy, fiber, and nutrients.

- Healthy Fats: Sources like avocados, nuts, seeds, and plant-based oils (olive, coconut) are included for essential fatty acids and fat-soluble vitamins.

- Minimized Animal Products: Animal products like meat, dairy, and eggs are limited or excluded, though some variations of a plant-based diet might include occasional consumption of these items.

Types of Plant-Based Diets

- Vegan: Strictly avoids all animal products, including meat, dairy, eggs, and often excludes other animal-derived products like honey.

- Vegetarian: Excludes meat but might include dairy products and eggs.

- Flexitarian/Semi-Vegetarian: Primarily plant-based but occasionally includes small amounts of meat, fish, or poultry.

- Pescatarian: Mostly plant-based with the inclusion of fish but excludes other meats.

Health Benefits of a Plant-Based Diet:

- Heart Health: High intake of fruits, vegetables, and fiber can lower the risk of heart disease by reducing cholesterol levels and blood pressure.

- Weight Management: Plant-based diets tend to be lower in calories and saturated fats, potentially aiding in weight loss and maintenance.

- Improved Digestion: Higher fiber content in plant-based foods promotes digestive health and helps prevent constipation.

- Lower Risk of Chronic Diseases: Studies suggest that plant-based diets may lower the risk of certain cancers, diabetes, and hypertension.

- Environmental Sustainability: Plant-based diets generally have a lower environmental impact, requiring fewer resources like water and land compared to animal agriculture.

Potential Concerns and Considerations

- Nutrient Deficiencies: While plant-based diets offer many nutrients, some may need to be mindful of obtaining enough protein, calcium, iron, vitamin B12, and omega-3 fatty acids, which can be less abundant in plant sources.

- Planning and Variety: It's crucial to plan meals to ensure a well-rounded intake of nutrients and variety in food choices.

- Social and Practical Challenges: Dining out or attending social events might pose challenges due to limited plant-based options.

Practical Tips for a Plant-Based Diet

- Gradual Transition: Start by gradually incorporating more plant-based meals into your diet rather than an abrupt change.

- Explore New Foods: Experiment with various plant-based ingredients and recipes to discover new flavors and textures.

- Education and Planning: Learn about nutrient-dense plant foods and plan meals to ensure a balanced intake of essential nutrients.

- Supplementation if Necessary: Consider supplements like vitamin B12 if certain nutrients are lacking in the diet.

Environmental impact and sustainability aspects

The environmental impact and sustainability of a plant-based diet have become increasingly significant in a world facing ecological challenges. Transitioning toward plant-based eating can significantly influence several facets of sustainability, including land and water use, greenhouse gas emissions, biodiversity conservation, and overall ecological balance.

Environmental Impact of Plant-Based Diets

- Land Use

Plant-based diets generally require less land compared to animal agriculture. Livestock farming demands vast areas for grazing and growing feed crops, contributing to deforestation and habitat destruction. By contrast, growing plant foods directly for human consumption uses land more efficiently, potentially reducing the overall demand for agricultural land.

- Water Usage

Animal agriculture is water-intensive, requiring vast amounts of water for livestock drinking, irrigation of feed crops, and processing. A shift to plant-based diets reduces water usage since most plant foods consume significantly less water during production compared to raising animals.

- Greenhouse Gas Emissions

Livestock farming is a major contributor to greenhouse gas emissions, particularly methane and nitrous oxide. Methane, emitted during digestion in ruminant animals like cows, has a high global warming potential. Plant-based diets, especially when avoiding or reducing animal products, can significantly decrease these emissions, mitigating the impact on climate change.

- Biodiversity Conservation

Animal agriculture is linked to biodiversity loss due to habitat destruction for grazing, monoculture feed crop production, and pollution. Choosing plant-based foods encourages more diverse and sustainable agricultural practices, reducing the pressure on ecosystems and promoting biodiversity conservation.

Sustainability Aspects of Plant-Based Diets

Reduced Environmental Footprint

Plant-based diets generally have a lower environmental impact compared to diets rich in animal products. Consuming plant-based foods requires fewer resources like water, land, and energy, contributing to a more sustainable food system.

- Mitigation of Deforestation

Animal agriculture, especially for grazing land and feed crop production, drives deforestation in many regions. Transitioning to plant-based diets reduces the demand for land and can help mitigate deforestation, preserving vital ecosystems and carbon sinks.

- Efficient Resource Use

Plant-based diets utilize resources more efficiently. Plants directly consumed by humans convert energy more effectively than growing crops for animal feed, thereby reducing the overall ecological footprint.

- Climate Change Mitigation

Reducing the consumption of animal products decreases greenhouse gas emissions associated with livestock farming. This mitigation effort aligns with global goals to combat climate change, contributing to a more sustainable future.

Challenges and Considerations

- Nutritional Adequacy

While plant-based diets offer numerous health benefits, ensuring adequate intake of certain nutrients like protein, iron, calcium, vitamin B12, and omega-3 fatty acids might require careful planning or supplementation.

- Access and Affordability

Access to a diverse range of plant-based foods and their affordability can be challenging in certain regions or socioeconomic contexts, potentially hindering widespread adoption of plant-based diets.

- Cultural and Social Factors

Cultural traditions, social norms, and personal preferences often influence dietary choices. Transitioning to a plant-based diet may face resistance or challenges due to these factors.

Promoting Sustainability Through Plant-Based Diets

- Education and Awareness

Raising awareness about the environmental impact of dietary choices can encourage individuals and communities to adopt more sustainable eating habits.

- Policy Support

Government policies supporting sustainable agriculture, promoting plant-based food availability, and incentivizing eco-friendly practices can facilitate the transition to more sustainable diets.

- Consumer Choices and Behavior Change

Encouraging and promoting plant-based diets through campaigns, educational programs, and initiatives can influence consumer choices and foster a shift towards more sustainable eating patterns.

The environmental impact and sustainability aspects of plant-based diets are substantial. Transitioning towards plant-based eating can significantly reduce environmental degradation, conserve natural resources, mitigate climate change, and promote a more sustainable food system. However, addressing challenges related to nutritional adequacy, accessibility, affordability, and cultural factors is crucial for a successful and widespread adoption of plant-based diets.

Efforts from individuals, communities, policymakers, and the food industry are essential to support and promote the sustainability benefits of plant-based eating for a healthier planet.

Tips for transitioning gradually or making an immediate switch

Transitioning to a plant-based diet is a commendable choice that can bring numerous health and environmental benefits. Whether you're considering a gradual shift or an immediate switch, it's essential to approach this change thoughtfully to ensure it's sustainable and meets your nutritional needs.

Understanding a Plant-Based Diet

A plant-based diet emphasizes whole, plant-derived foods while minimizing or eliminating animal products. It primarily consists of fruits, vegetables, whole grains, legumes, nuts, and seeds. To transition successfully, consider the following steps:

Gradual Transition

Transitioning gradually can help your body adjust and make the process more sustainable.

1. Educate Yourself

Start by learning about plant-based nutrition. Understand essential nutrients like protein, iron, calcium, vitamin B12, and omega-3 fatty acids. Recognize plant-based sources for these nutrients to ensure a balanced diet.

2. Incremental Changes

Begin by incorporating more plant-based meals into your routine. Start with one meal a day or dedicate specific days in a week to plant-based eating. Gradually increase the frequency as you become comfortable.

3. Experiment with Recipes

Explore diverse plant-based recipes to find meals that appeal to your taste buds. Experiment with different cuisines and cooking methods to keep your meals exciting and satisfying.

4. Focus on Whole Foods

Emphasize whole foods like fruits, vegetables, whole grains, legumes, nuts, and seeds rather than relying on processed plant-based alternatives. Whole foods offer more nutrients and health benefits.

5. Monitor Nutrient Intake

Track your nutrient intake, especially when transitioning, to ensure you're meeting your body's needs. Consider consulting a dietitian or nutritionist for personalized guidance.

Immediate Switch

An immediate transition requires more commitment and planning to ensure a smooth adjustment.

1. Planning & Preparation

Before making the switch, plan your meals for the upcoming days or weeks. Stock up on a variety of plant-based foods to avoid feeling deprived or overwhelmed.

2. Replace Animal Products

Replace animal-based foods in your diet with plant-based alternatives. For example, switch from cow's milk to almond, soy, or oat milk, and use tofu or tempeh instead of meat in your dishes.

3. Explore Plant-Based Proteins

Experiment with various plant-based protein sources such as lentils, beans, chickpeas, quinoa, and edamame. These can be incorporated into salads, soups, stir-fries, and more.

4. Stay Mindful of Nutrients

Pay attention to essential nutrients initially, ensuring you're getting enough iron, calcium, protein, and vitamins. Consider taking supplements if needed, especially vitamin B12.

5. Find Support

Seek support from friends, online communities, or local groups following a plant-based lifestyle. Sharing experiences and tips can be immensely helpful during this transition.

General Tips for Both Approaches

- Variety is Key: Aim for a diverse range of plant-based foods to ensure a wide array of nutrients.

- Read Labels: Be mindful of hidden animal-derived ingredients in packaged foods.

- Stay Hydrated: Drink an adequate amount of water and consider herbal teas or infused water for variety.

- Mindful Eating: Focus on mindful eating, savoring each bite and paying attention to your body's hunger and fullness cues.

- Be Patient: Give your body time to adjust. Digestive changes or cravings for familiar foods are normal during the transition period.

How to ensure nutritional adequacy and balance in a plant-based diet

Ensuring nutritional adequacy and balance in a plant-based diet is crucial for maintaining optimal health. While a plant-based diet offers numerous benefits, it requires thoughtful planning to ensure you obtain all essential nutrients. Here's an exploration of key nutrients and strategies to achieve nutritional balance:

Essential Nutrients in a Plant-Based Diet

1. Protein

Plant-based sources of protein include legumes (beans, lentils), tofu, tempeh, seitan, edamame, quinoa, nuts, and seeds. Combining different protein sources throughout the day ensures a variety of amino acids, building blocks of protein.

2. Iron

Plant-based iron sources include lentils, chickpeas, tofu, spinach, fortified cereals, pumpkin seeds, and quinoa. Consuming vitamin C-rich foods alongside iron-rich foods aids iron absorption.

3. Calcium

Calcium sources in a plant-based diet include fortified plant milks, tofu, almonds, leafy greens (kale, collard greens), and fortified orange juice. Ensuring an adequate intake of calcium-rich foods is essential for bone health.

4. Vitamin B12

Vitamin B12 is primarily found in animal products. Fortified foods like nutritional yeast, fortified plant milks, and B12 supplements are necessary for those following a plant-based diet to avoid deficiency.

5. Omega-3 Fatty Acids

Sources include flaxseeds, chia seeds, hemp seeds, walnuts, and algae-based supplements. Omega-3s are crucial for heart and brain health.

6. Zinc

Plant-based zinc sources include legumes, nuts, seeds, whole grains, and fortified cereals. Consuming these foods regularly helps maintain adequate zinc levels.

Strategies for Nutritional Adequacy in a Plant-Based Diet

1. Diverse Diet

Consume a wide variety of plant-based foods to ensure a broad spectrum of nutrients. Rotate vegetables, fruits, legumes, whole grains, nuts, and seeds to maximize nutrient intake.

2. Fortified Foods

Incorporate fortified plant milks, cereals, and nutritional yeast to supplement nutrients like calcium, vitamin B12, and vitamin D.

3. Balanced Meals

Ensure each meal comprises a combination of carbohydrates, proteins, healthy fats, and a variety of colorful fruits and vegetables to obtain a range of nutrients.

4. Monitor Portion Sizes

Maintain portion sizes to avoid excessive calorie intake while ensuring a balanced distribution of nutrients throughout the day.

5. Nutrient-Rich Snacks

Opt for nutrient-dense snacks like nuts, seeds, fruits, or veggie sticks with hummus to supplement your nutrient intake between meals.

6. Consider Supplements

Consult a healthcare professional to assess if you need supplements, especially for vitamin B12, vitamin D, or omega-3 fatty acids.

Sample Meal Plan for Nutritional Balance

Breakfast

Overnight oats made with almond milk, topped with mixed berries, chia seeds, and a sprinkle of almonds.

A glass of fortified orange juice for added vitamin C.

Snack

Carrot sticks with hummus or a handful of mixed nuts and seeds.

Lunch

Quinoa salad with mixed greens, chickpeas, cherry tomatoes, cucumber, and a tahini-lemon dressing.

A side of sautéed kale for added calcium.

Snack

A smoothie made with spinach, banana, flaxseeds, and plant-based protein powder.

Dinner

Stir-fried tofu and vegetable medley (bell peppers, broccoli, snap peas) served with brown rice.

A side of steamed edamame for extra protein.

Additional Tips for Nutritional Balance:

1. Read Labels

Check food labels for added nutrients and ensure they align with your dietary needs.

2. Cooking Methods

Opt for steaming, baking, or sautéing instead of deep-frying to retain the maximum nutritional value of foods.

3. Hydration

Stay adequately hydrated by drinking water or herbal teas throughout the day.

4. Listen to Your Body

Pay attention to your body's cues. If you feel fatigued or notice any unusual symptoms, consult a healthcare professional.

5. Seek Professional Guidance

Consider consulting a registered dietitian or nutritionist experienced in plant-based nutrition to create a personalized plan that meets your specific nutritional needs.

Navigating restaurants and social gatherings as a plant-based eater

Navigating restaurants and social gatherings as a plant-based eater can be both exciting and challenging. While it's a chance to explore new culinary experiences and share your dietary choices with others, it might also present situations where finding suitable options or dealing with social dynamics can be tricky. Here's a comprehensive guide on how to navigate these scenarios successfully:

Restaurants

1. Research and Choose Wisely:

Before dining out, research restaurants with plant-based options. Many establishments now have dedicated plant-based menus or items marked as vegetarian/vegan.

2. Call Ahead:

Call the restaurant in advance to inquire about their plant-based offerings or to request modifications to existing dishes. This ensures they can accommodate your dietary preferences.

3. Customize Your Order:

Don't hesitate to ask for modifications to suit your plant-based needs. For example, ask for substitutions or omissions of certain ingredients.

4. Be Clear with Servers:

Communicate your dietary requirements clearly to the server. Specify that you're vegan or vegetarian to avoid misunderstandings.

5. Flexibility:

Be open to adapting dishes or creating custom meals based on available ingredients. Many restaurants are willing to accommodate requests if you're flexible.

Social Gatherings:

1. Communicate in Advance:

Inform the host or organizer about your dietary preferences beforehand. Offer to bring a plant-based dish to share, ensuring there's something you can eat.

2. Offer Assistance:

Offer to help prepare meals or suggest plant-based recipes that could complement the gathering's menu. It can be an opportunity to introduce others to delicious plant-based options.

3. Be Prepared:

If attending a potluck or event where food options might be limited, eat something beforehand to ensure you're not hungry and have a backup plan.

4. Educate Without Being Overbearing:

If asked about your dietary choice, share your reasons politely without imposing your beliefs. Be open to answering questions but avoid preaching or making others uncomfortable.

5. Focus on Enjoying the Company:

While food is often a centerpiece of social gatherings, prioritize enjoying the company of friends or family rather than solely focusing on the menu.

Tips for Various Scenarios:

- **Casual Dining**

Opt for restaurants with diverse menu options, such as Mexican, Middle Eastern, or Asian cuisines, which often have plant-based choices like veggie burritos, falafel, or tofu stir-fries.

- **Formal Dining**

Call ahead to upscale restaurants to discuss dietary preferences and ensure they can accommodate your needs. Look for gourmet plant-based options or request modifications to existing dishes.

- **Fast Food**

Some fast-food chains now offer plant-based alternatives. Look for veggie burgers, salads, or customizable options that fit your dietary requirements.

- **Traveling**

Research local eateries or use apps/websites that cater to plant-based dining to find suitable restaurants or grocery stores with plant-based options.

Maintaining Social Ease

1. Confidence in Your Choices

Be confident in your dietary choices without feeling the need to justify or explain them extensively. Own your decision with pride.

2. Bring Snacks

Carry portable plant-based snacks like nuts, fruit, energy bars, or trail mix in case you can't find suitable options while out.

3. Share the Experience

If dining with non-plant-based eaters, encourage sharing dishes to introduce them to your favorite plant-based options. It fosters a communal dining experience.

4. Stay Positive

Approach dining out or social gatherings with a positive attitude. Focus on the available options rather than feeling restricted by limitations.

5. Be Grateful and Appreciative

Express gratitude when hosts or restaurants accommodate your dietary needs. Positive feedback encourages them to continue offering plant-based options.

Navigating restaurants and social gatherings as a plant-based eater involves a combination of planning, communication, flexibility, and confidence. By researching options beforehand, communicating clearly, offering assistance, and staying open-minded, you can enjoy delicious plant-based meals while fostering positive interactions in various social settings. Remember, your dietary choices are a part of who you are, and approaching them with confidence and grace can positively influence those around you.

Addressing concerns about protein, energy, and performance

A plant-based diet has gained traction for its health benefits and sustainability. However, concerns often arise about meeting protein needs, sustaining energy levels, and maintaining optimal performance without animal products.

Addressing these concerns requires a comprehensive understanding of nutritional principles and strategic dietary planning.

Protein is a crucial macronutrient necessary for various bodily functions, including muscle repair and immune system support. Concerns about inadequate protein intake on a plant-based diet are prevalent due to the perception that animal products are superior protein sources. However, numerous plant-based foods offer ample protein. Legumes like lentils, chickpeas, and beans, along with tofu, tempeh, quinoa, and nuts, are rich sources of plant-based protein. Combining different plant protein sources throughout the day ensures a diverse amino acid profile, fulfilling the body's needs for essential amino acids.

Moreover, protein complementation, the strategic pairing of different plant-based protein sources, allows for a balanced intake of essential amino acids. For instance, combining beans with rice or lentils with seeds forms complete protein sources. Additionally, fortified foods like certain plant-based milks and cereals contribute to meeting daily protein requirements.

Energy levels play a pivotal role in maintaining vitality and overall well-being. Concerns arise regarding plant-based diets' ability to provide sustained energy due to misconceptions about insufficient calorie intake or deficiencies in certain nutrients. However, when appropriately planned, plant-based diets can offer abundant energy through nutrient-dense foods.

Whole grains like quinoa, brown rice, oats, and whole-grain bread provide complex carbohydrates, supplying a steady release of energy. Incorporating a variety of fruits and vegetables ensures an intake of essential vitamins, minerals, and antioxidants, vital for energy production and overall health. Furthermore, healthy fats from sources like avocados, nuts, seeds, and olive oil contribute to satiety and sustained energy levels.

Strategic meal planning is pivotal in ensuring a well-rounded plant-based diet that meets energy requirements. Balancing meals with a variety of whole foods from different food groups helps maintain energy levels throughout the day. Snacking on nuts, seeds, or fruits can also provide quick energy boosts without relying on processed or high-sugar snacks.

Optimal performance, whether in athletics or daily activities, is a concern for those transitioning to or maintaining a plant-based lifestyle. The misconception that animal products are essential for peak performance persists, but numerous athletes thriving on plant-based diets debunk this belief.

Athletes can meet their increased energy and nutrient needs through a well-designed plant-based diet. Adequate carbohydrate intake from whole grains, fruits, and vegetables supports glycogen stores, essential for sustained physical performance. Plant-based protein sources, coupled with careful planning to ensure sufficient intake, facilitate muscle repair and recovery.

Additionally, incorporating iron-rich foods like legumes, tofu, spinach, and fortified cereals aids in preventing anemia, which can impact performance. Vitamin B12 supplementation is crucial for plant-based individuals as this vitamin is predominantly found in animal products; it plays a pivotal role in energy production and nerve function.

Moreover, plant-based diets can contribute to faster recovery due to their anti-inflammatory properties derived from high antioxidant content. Foods like turmeric, berries, and leafy greens possess anti-inflammatory effects, potentially reducing muscle soreness and enhancing overall recovery post-exercise.

Concerns about protein adequacy, sustained energy levels, and optimal performance on a plant-based diet can be effectively addressed through strategic dietary planning. Emphasizing a diverse range of plant-based protein sources, complementation of amino acids, and careful consideration of nutrient-dense foods ensure meeting protein needs.

Balancing meals with complex carbohydrates, healthy fats, and a variety of fruits and vegetables sustains energy levels throughout the day. Athletes and individuals seeking optimal performance can thrive on a plant-based diet by ensuring sufficient intake of key nutrients, including carbohydrates, proteins, iron, B12, and antioxidants, while also capitalizing on the diet's potential for faster recovery and reduced inflammation.

Ultimately, education, mindful planning, and a diverse selection of plant-based foods empower individuals to thrive physically and perform optimally while embracing a plant-centric lifestyle.

Chapter 2

Breakfast

Vegan Pancakes

Preparation time: 10 minutes

Cooking time: 15 minutes

Number of servings: 4

Ingredients:

- 1 cup all-purpose flour

- 1 tablespoon sugar

- 2 teaspoons baking powder

- 1/4 teaspoon salt

- 1 cup almond milk (or any plant-based milk)

- 2 tablespoons melted coconut oil (or vegetable oil)

- 1 teaspoon vanilla extract

Directions:

1. In a mixing bowl, whisk together the flour, sugar, baking powder, and salt.

2. In a separate bowl, combine the almond milk, melted coconut oil, and vanilla extract.

3. Pour the wet ingredients into the dry ingredients and stir until just combined. Do not overmix; a few lumps are okay.

4. Heat a non-stick skillet or griddle over medium heat. Lightly grease the surface with oil or cooking spray.

5. Pour 1/4 cup of batter onto the skillet for each pancake. Cook until bubbles form on the surface, then flip and cook the other side until golden brown.

6. Repeat with the remaining batter.

7. Serve warm with your favorite toppings like maple syrup, fresh fruits, or dairy-free whipped cream.

Nutritional info: (per serving, without toppings)

- Calories: 220

- Fat: 8g

- Carbohydrates: 32g

- Protein: 4g

- Fiber: 1g

Chia Seed Pudding

Preparation time: 5 minutes (plus chilling time)

Cooking time: 0 minutes

Number of servings: 2

Ingredients:

- 1/4 cup chia seeds

- 1 cup almond milk (or any plant-based milk)

- 1 tablespoon maple syrup (or sweetener of choice)

- 1/2 teaspoon vanilla extract

- Toppings: fresh berries, sliced fruits, nuts, shredded coconut

Directions:

1. In a bowl or jar, combine chia seeds, almond milk, maple syrup, and vanilla extract. Mix well.

2. Cover the bowl or jar and refrigerate for at least 2 hours or overnight.

3. Stir the mixture after the first 10 minutes to prevent clumping and then again before leaving it to chill.

4. Once the pudding has thickened to your desired consistency, serve it in bowls or jars.

5. Add your favorite toppings like fresh berries, sliced fruits, nuts, or shredded coconut.

6. Enjoy your creamy and nutritious chia seed pudding!

Nutritional info: (per serving, without toppings)

- Calories: 150

- Fat: 8g

- Carbohydrates: 14g

- Protein: 5g

- Fiber: 9g

Tofu Scramble

Preparation time: 10 minutes

Cooking time: 10 minutes

Number of servings: 2-3

Ingredients:

- 1 block (14-16 oz) firm tofu, drained and pressed

- 2 tablespoons nutritional yeast

- 1/2 teaspoon turmeric powder

- 1/2 teaspoon garlic powder

- 1/2 teaspoon onion powder

- Salt and pepper to taste

- 1 tablespoon olive oil

- Optional add-ins: diced vegetables (bell peppers, onions, spinach), vegan cheese, chopped tomatoes

Directions:

1. Heat olive oil in a skillet over medium heat.

2. Crumble the pressed tofu into the skillet, resembling scrambled eggs.

3. Sprinkle nutritional yeast, turmeric powder, garlic powder, onion powder, salt, and pepper over the tofu.

4. Mix well to evenly distribute the seasonings.

5. Cook for about 5-7 minutes, stirring occasionally.

6. If adding vegetables, toss them in and cook until they soften.

7. Adjust seasoning to taste and add any optional add-ins like vegan cheese or chopped tomatoes.

8. Serve hot with toast or alongside your favorite breakfast sides.

Nutritional info: (per serving, without add-ins)

- Calories: 180

- Fat: 10g

- Carbohydrates: 5g

- Protein: 20g

- Fiber: 2g

Smoothie Bowl

Preparation time: 5 minutes

Cooking time: 0 minutes

Number of servings: 1

Ingredients:

- 1 frozen banana

- 1/2 cup frozen mixed berries

- 1/2 cup spinach or kale

- 1/2 cup almond milk (or any plant-based milk)

- Toppings: granola, sliced fruits, shredded coconut, chia seeds, nuts

Directions:

1. In a blender, combine the frozen banana, frozen berries, spinach or kale, and almond milk.

2. Blend until smooth and creamy, adding more liquid if needed to reach your desired consistency.

3. Pour the smoothie into a bowl.

4. Top the smoothie bowl with granola, sliced fruits, shredded coconut, chia seeds, nuts, or any other desired toppings.

5. Serve immediately and enjoy your nutritious smoothie bowl!

Nutritional info: (without toppings)

- Calories: 200

- Fat: 2g

- Carbohydrates: 45g

- Protein: 3g

- Fiber: 8g

Breakfast Burrito with Beans and Veggies

Preparation time: 15 minutes

Cooking time: 10 minutes

Number of servings: 2-3

Ingredients:

- 4 large tortillas

- 1 can (15 oz) black beans, drained and rinsed

- 1 cup diced bell peppers (any color)

- 1 cup diced onions

- 1 cup diced tomatoes

- 1 cup chopped spinach or kale

- 1 teaspoon cumin powder

- 1 teaspoon paprika

- Salt and pepper to taste

- 1 tablespoon olive oil

- Optional toppings: avocado slices, salsa, vegan cheese, cilantro

Directions:

1. Heat olive oil in a skillet over medium heat.

2. Add diced onions and bell peppers to the skillet. Sauté until they soften.

3. Add black beans, diced tomatoes, chopped spinach or kale, cumin powder, paprika, salt, and pepper. Mix well and cook for a few minutes until heated through.

4. Warm the tortillas in a separate skillet or microwave.

5. Place a generous amount of the bean and veggie mixture onto each tortilla.

6. Add optional toppings like avocado slices, salsa, vegan cheese, or cilantro if desired.

7. Roll the tortillas tightly into burritos.

8. Serve immediately and enjoy your flavorful breakfast burritos!

Nutritional info: (per serving, without optional toppings)

- Calories: 380

- Fat: 8g

- Carbohydrates: 63g

- Protein: 15g

- Fiber: 16g

Vegan Breakfast Tacos

Preparation time: 15 minutes

Cooking time: 10 minutes

Number of servings: 2-3

Ingredients:

- 6 small corn tortillas

- 1 block (14-16 oz) firm tofu, drained and pressed

- 1/2 teaspoon turmeric powder

- 1/2 teaspoon garlic powder

- 1/2 teaspoon onion powder

- Salt and pepper to taste

- 1 tablespoon olive oil

- Toppings: sliced avocado, salsa, chopped cilantro, lime wedges

Directions:

1. Crumble the pressed tofu into a bowl.

2. Heat olive oil in a skillet over medium heat.

3. Add the crumbled tofu to the skillet.

4. Sprinkle turmeric powder, garlic powder, onion powder, salt, and pepper over the tofu. Mix well.

5. Cook for about 5-7 minutes, stirring occasionally.

6. Warm the corn tortillas in a separate skillet or microwave.

7. Spoon the tofu scramble onto each tortilla.

8. Add toppings like sliced avocado, salsa, chopped cilantro, or a squeeze of lime juice.

9. Serve warm and enjoy your delicious vegan breakfast tacos! Nutritional info: (per serving, without toppings)

- Calories: 250

- Fat: 10g

- Carbohydrates: 28g

- Protein: 14g

- Fiber: 5g

Quinoa Breakfast Bowl

Preparation time: 15 minutes

Cooking time: 15 minutes

Number of servings: 2

Ingredients:

- 1 cup cooked quinoa

- 1 cup diced sweet potatoes

- 1 cup black beans, cooked or canned, drained and rinsed

- 1 cup chopped kale or spinach

- 1/2 teaspoon smoked paprika

- 1/2 teaspoon garlic powder

- Salt and pepper to taste

- 2 tablespoons olive oil

- Optional toppings: sliced avocado, hot sauce, chopped green onions

Directions:

1. Heat olive oil in a skillet over medium heat.

2. Add diced sweet potatoes to the skillet and cook until they soften, about 8-10 minutes.

3. Add black beans, chopped kale or spinach, smoked paprika, garlic powder, salt, and pepper. Mix well and cook for a few more minutes until everything is heated through.

4. Divide the cooked quinoa between two bowls.

5. Top the quinoa with the sweet potato and black bean mixture.

6. Add optional toppings like sliced avocado, hot sauce, or chopped green onions.

7. Serve warm and enjoy your nourishing quinoa breakfast bowl! Nutritional info: (per serving, without optional toppings)

- Calories: 380

- Fat: 12g

- Carbohydrates: 55g

- Protein: 15g

- Fiber: 13g

Vegan French Toast

Preparation time: 10 minutes

Cooking time: 10 minutes

Number of servings: 2-3

Ingredients:

- 6 slices of thick bread (preferably day-old bread)

- 1 cup unsweetened almond milk (or any plant-based milk)

- 2 tablespoons flour

- 1 tablespoon nutritional yeast

- 1 tablespoon maple syrup

- 1 teaspoon vanilla extract

- 1/2 teaspoon ground cinnamon

- Pinch of salt

- Vegan butter or oil for frying

- Optional toppings: fresh fruits, maple syrup, powdered sugar

Directions:

1. In a shallow dish, whisk together almond milk, flour, nutritional yeast, maple syrup, vanilla extract, ground cinnamon, and a pinch of salt until well combined.

2. Heat a skillet or griddle over medium heat and add vegan butter or a little oil to coat the surface.

3. Dip each slice of bread into the batter, coating both sides evenly.

4. Place the coated bread slices onto the heated skillet or griddle.

5. Cook for 3-4 minutes on each side, or until golden brown and slightly crispy.

6. Remove from the skillet and serve hot.

7. Top with fresh fruits, a drizzle of maple syrup, or a sprinkle of powdered sugar if desired.

8. Enjoy your delicious vegan French toast!

Nutritional info: (per serving, without toppings)

- Calories: 250

- Fat: 5g

- Carbohydrates: 45g

- Protein: 8g

- Fiber: 4g

Acai Bowl

Preparation time: 10 minutes

Cooking time: 0 minutes

Number of servings: 1

Ingredients:

- 1 packet frozen unsweetened acai puree (100g), or 1/2 cup acai puree

- 1 frozen banana

- 1/2 cup frozen mixed berries

- 1/2 cup almond milk (or any plant-based milk)

- Toppings: granola, sliced fruits, shredded coconut, chia seeds, nuts, honey or agave syrup (optional)

Directions:

1. In a blender, combine the frozen acai puree, frozen banana, frozen mixed berries, and almond milk.

2. Blend until smooth and creamy, adding more liquid if needed to achieve a thick smoothie consistency.

3. Pour the blended acai mixture into a bowl.

4. Top the acai bowl with granola, sliced fruits, shredded coconut, chia seeds, nuts, and a drizzle of honey or agave syrup if desired.

5. Serve immediately and enjoy your refreshing acai bowl!

Nutritional info: (without toppings)

- Calories: 250

- Fat: 5g

- Carbohydrates: 45g

- Protein: 4g

- Fiber: 8g

Sweet Potato Hash

Preparation time: 15 minutes

Cooking time: 20 minutes

Number of servings: 2-3

Ingredients:

- 2 medium sweet potatoes, peeled and diced

- 1 bell pepper, diced

- 1 onion, diced

- 2 cloves garlic, minced

- 1 teaspoon smoked paprika

- 1/2 teaspoon cumin

- Salt and pepper to taste

- 2 tablespoons olive oil

- Fresh parsley or cilantro for garnish (optional)

Directions:

1. Heat olive oil in a skillet over medium-high heat.

2. Add diced sweet potatoes to the skillet and cook for about 8-10 minutes, stirring occasionally, until they start to soften.

3. Add diced bell pepper, onion, and minced garlic to the skillet. Cook for another 5-7 minutes, or until the vegetables are tender.

4. Sprinkle smoked paprika, cumin, salt, and pepper over the sweet potato mixture. Stir well to combine and cook for an additional 2-3 minutes.

5. Adjust seasoning if needed and remove from heat.

6. Serve the sweet potato hash hot, garnished with fresh parsley or cilantro if desired.

7. Enjoy your flavorful and hearty sweet potato hash!

   Nutritional info: (per serving)

- Calories: 220

- Fat: 7g

- Carbohydrates: 36g

- Protein: 4g

- Fiber: 6g

Vegan Breakfast Sandwich

Preparation time: 10 minutes

Cooking time: 10 minutes

Number of servings: 2

Ingredients:

- 4 slices of whole grain bread or English muffins

- 1 block (14-16 oz) firm tofu, drained and pressed

- 1/2 teaspoon turmeric powder

- 1/2 teaspoon garlic powder

- 1/2 teaspoon onion powder

- Salt and pepper to taste

- Vegan cheese slices (optional)

- Vegan mayo or avocado slices

- Sliced tomatoes, lettuce, or spinach

Directions:

1. Slice the tofu into even pieces (similar to the size of the bread slices).

2. In a bowl, mix turmeric powder, garlic powder, onion powder, salt, and pepper.

3. Sprinkle the spice mix evenly over the tofu slices, coating both sides.

4. Heat a skillet over medium heat and lightly oil the surface.

5. Cook the tofu slices for about 3-4 minutes on each side, or until golden brown and slightly crispy.

6. If using vegan cheese, place a slice on each tofu piece in the last minute of cooking to melt.

7. Toast the whole grain bread slices or English muffins.

8. Assemble the sandwiches: spread vegan mayo or avocado on one side of each slice, add tofu slices, sliced tomatoes, lettuce or spinach, and any other desired toppings.

9. Put together the sandwiches and serve immediately.

10. Enjoy your flavorful vegan breakfast sandwiches!

    Nutritional info: (per serving, without optional toppings)

- Calories: 320

- Fat: 14g

- Carbohydrates: 30g

- Protein: 18g

- Fiber: 6g

Fruit Salad with Nuts and Seeds

Preparation time: 10 minutes

Cooking time: 0 minutes

Number of servings: 4

Ingredients:

- 2 cups mixed fresh fruits (such as strawberries, blueberries, pineapple, mango, kiwi)

- 1/4 cup chopped nuts (almonds, walnuts, or pecans)

- 2 tablespoons mixed seeds (chia seeds, pumpkin seeds, sunflower seeds)

- Optional: fresh mint leaves for garnish

Dressing:

- 2 tablespoons maple syrup or honey (if not strictly vegan)

- 1 tablespoon lime juice

- Zest of 1 lime

- Pinch of cinnamon

Directions:

1. Wash and chop the fresh fruits into bite-sized pieces if needed.

2. In a bowl, combine the mixed fruits, chopped nuts, and mixed
    seeds.

3. In a separate small bowl, whisk together the maple syrup or
    honey, lime juice, lime zest, and a pinch of cinnamon to make
    the dressing.

4. Drizzle the dressing over the fruit, nuts, and seed mixture.

5. Gently toss everything together until well coated.

6. Garnish with fresh mint leaves if desired.

7. Serve the fruit salad immediately or refrigerate until ready to
    serve.

8. Enjoy your refreshing and nutritious fruit salad!

    Nutritional info: (per serving)

- Calories: 150

- Fat: 8g

- Carbohydrates: 20g

- Protein: 3g

- Fiber: 4g

Vegan Breakfast Casserole

Preparation time: 15 minutes

Cooking time: 40 minutes

Number of servings: 6

Ingredients:

- 1 block (14-16 oz) firm tofu, drained and pressed

- 1 cup diced bell peppers (any color)

- 1 cup diced onions

- 2 cups chopped spinach or kale

- 1 cup cherry tomatoes, halved

- 1 teaspoon garlic powder

- 1 teaspoon onion powder

- 1/2 teaspoon turmeric powder

- Salt and pepper to taste

- 1 tablespoon nutritional yeast (optional)

- 2 tablespoons olive oil

Directions:

1. Preheat the oven to 375°F (190°C).

2. In a skillet, heat olive oil over medium heat.

3. Add diced onions and bell peppers. Sauté until they soften.

4. Crumble the pressed tofu into the skillet.

5. Add garlic powder, onion powder, turmeric powder, salt, and pepper. Mix well.

6. Cook for about 5 minutes, stirring occasionally.

7. Add chopped spinach or kale, and halved cherry tomatoes. Cook for another 2-3 minutes until the greens wilt slightly.

8. If using nutritional yeast, stir it in for added flavor.

9. Transfer the tofu and vegetable mixture to a greased baking dish.

10. Spread it evenly in the dish.

11. Bake for 25-30 minutes until the top is slightly golden.

12. Remove from the oven and let it cool for a few minutes before slicing.

13. Serve warm and enjoy your delicious vegan breakfast casserole!

Nutritional info: (per serving)

- Calories: 180

- Fat: 10g

- Carbohydrates: 10g

- Protein: 15g

- Fiber: 3g

Vegan Waffles

Preparation time: 10 minutes

Cooking time: 15 minutes

Number of servings: 4

Ingredients:

- 1 1/2 cups all-purpose flour

- 2 tablespoons sugar (or sweetener of choice)

- 2 teaspoons baking powder

- 1/2 teaspoon baking soda

- 1/4 teaspoon salt

- 1 3/4 cups almond milk (or any plant-based milk)

- 1/4 cup melted coconut oil (or vegetable oil)

- 1 teaspoon vanilla extract

Directions:

1. Preheat your waffle iron according to its instructions.

2. In a large mixing bowl, whisk together the flour, sugar, baking powder, baking soda, and salt.

3. In another bowl, combine almond milk, melted coconut oil, and vanilla extract.

4. Pour the wet ingredients into the dry ingredients and whisk until just combined. Do not overmix; a few lumps are okay.

5. Lightly grease the waffle iron if needed.

6. Ladle the batter onto the waffle iron and cook according to the manufacturer's instructions or until golden and crisp.

7. Repeat with the remaining batter.

8. Serve the waffles warm with your favorite toppings like fresh fruit, maple syrup, or dairy-free whipped cream.

Nutritional info: (per serving, without toppings)

- Calories: 280

- Fat: 12g

- Carbohydrates: 38g

- Protein: 5g

- Fiber: 1g

Oatmeal with Berries and Nuts

Preparation time: 5 minutes

Cooking time: 5 minutes

Number of servings: 2

Ingredients:

- 1 cup rolled oats

- 2 cups water or plant-based milk

- 1/2 cup mixed berries (strawberries, blueberries, raspberries)

- 1/4 cup chopped nuts (almonds, walnuts, or pecans)

- 2 tablespoons maple syrup or honey (if not strictly vegan)

- Pinch of cinnamon

- Optional toppings: sliced bananas, chia seeds, shredded coconut

Directions:

1. In a saucepan, bring water or plant-based milk to a boil.

2. Stir in the rolled oats and reduce the heat to medium-low.

3. Cook for about 3-5 minutes, stirring occasionally, until the oats reach your desired consistency.

4. Once cooked, remove the oats from heat and divide into serving bowls.

5. Top the oatmeal with mixed berries, chopped nuts, maple syrup or honey, a pinch of cinnamon, and any optional toppings you prefer.

6. Serve hot and enjoy your comforting oatmeal with berries and nuts!

Nutritional info: (per serving, without optional toppings)

- Calories: 300

- Fat: 10g

- Carbohydrates: 45g

- Protein: 8g

- Fiber: 7g

Vegan Breakfast Cookies

Preparation time: 15 minutes

Cooking time: 15 minutes

Number of servings: 12 cookies

Ingredients:

- 2 ripe bananas, mashed

- 1/4 cup almond butter (or any nut/seed butter)

- 1/4 cup maple syrup or agave syrup

- 1 teaspoon vanilla extract

- 1 1/2 cups rolled oats

- 1/2 cup shredded coconut

- 1/4 cup chopped nuts or seeds (almonds, walnuts, sunflower seeds)

- 1/4 cup dried fruits (raisins, cranberries, chopped dates)

Directions:

1. Preheat the oven to 350°F (175°C). Line a baking sheet with parchment paper.

2. In a mixing bowl, combine mashed bananas, almond butter, maple syrup or agave syrup, and vanilla extract. Mix until well combined.

3. Add rolled oats, shredded coconut, chopped nuts or seeds, and dried fruits to the wet mixture. Stir until everything is evenly combined and forms a sticky batter.

4. Scoop spoonfuls of the batter and drop them onto the prepared baking sheet, shaping them into cookie shapes.

5. Flatten the cookies slightly with the back of a spoon or your fingers.

6. Bake for 12-15 minutes or until the cookies turn golden brown around the edges.

7. Remove from the oven and let them cool on the baking sheet for a few minutes before transferring to a wire rack to cool completely.

8. Once cooled, store the vegan breakfast cookies in an airtight container.

Nutritional info: (per cookie)

- Calories: 120

- Fat: 6g

- Carbohydrates: 16g

- Protein: 3g

- Fiber: 2g

Veggie Frittata

Preparation time: 15 minutes

Cooking time: 25 minutes

Number of servings: 4

Ingredients:

- 8 large eggs (for a vegan version, use a tofu scramble from previous recipes)

- 1 cup chopped mixed vegetables (bell peppers, onions, spinach, mushrooms)

- 1/2 cup cherry tomatoes, halved

- 1/4 cup chopped fresh herbs (parsley, basil, or thyme)

- 1/4 cup dairy-free cheese (optional)

- Salt and pepper to taste

- 2 tablespoons olive oil

Directions:

1. Preheat the oven to 350°F (175°C).

2. In a mixing bowl, beat the eggs (or prepare the tofu scramble as mentioned in previous recipes).

3. Heat olive oil in an oven-safe skillet over medium heat.

4. Add the chopped mixed vegetables and sauté until they start to soften.

5. Pour the beaten eggs (or tofu scramble) into the skillet over the vegetables.

6. Arrange cherry tomato halves on top.

7. Sprinkle with chopped fresh herbs, dairy-free cheese (if using), salt, and pepper.

8. Cook on the stovetop for about 3-4 minutes until the edges start to set.

9. Transfer the skillet to the preheated oven and bake for 15-20 minutes until the frittata is set in the middle and lightly browned on top.

10. Remove from the oven and let it cool for a few minutes before slicing.

11. Serve warm or at room temperature.

    Nutritional info: (per serving)

- Calories: 180

- Fat: 12g

- Carbohydrates: 6g

- Protein: 13g

- Fiber: 2g

Vegan Breakfast Burrito Bowl

Preparation time: 15 minutes

Cooking time: 15 minutes

Number of servings: 2

Ingredients:

- 1 cup cooked quinoa

- 1 cup black beans, cooked or canned, drained and rinsed

- 1 avocado, sliced

- 1 cup salsa

- 1 cup chopped lettuce or spinach

- 1/2 cup corn kernels (cooked)

- 1/2 cup diced tomatoes

- 1/4 cup diced red onion

- Juice of 1 lime

- Salt and pepper to taste

- Optional toppings: chopped cilantro, sliced jalapeños, hot sauce

Directions:

1. In a bowl, mix cooked quinoa, black beans, corn kernels, diced tomatoes, diced red onion, lime juice, salt, and pepper.

2. Divide the quinoa and bean mixture into serving bowls.

3. Top each bowl with sliced avocado, salsa, chopped lettuce or spinach, and any optional toppings you prefer.

4. Serve immediately and enjoy your vibrant and flavorful vegan breakfast burrito bowl!

Nutritional info: (per serving)

- Calories: 380

- Fat: 15g

- Carbohydrates: 50g

- Protein: 12g

- Fiber: 14g

Breakfast Quinoa Porridge

Preparation time: 5 minutes

Cooking time: 15 minutes

Number of servings: 2

Ingredients:

- 1/2 cup quinoa, rinsed

- 1 cup almond milk (or any plant-based milk)

- 1/2 cup water

- 2 tablespoons maple syrup or agave syrup

- 1/2 teaspoon ground cinnamon

- Pinch of salt

- Toppings: sliced bananas, berries, chopped nuts, coconut flakes

Directions:

1. In a saucepan, combine quinoa, almond milk, water, maple syrup or agave syrup, ground cinnamon, and a pinch of salt.

2. Bring the mixture to a boil over medium-high heat.

3. Reduce the heat to low, cover, and simmer for about 15 minutes or until the quinoa is cooked and most of the liquid is absorbed.

4. Stir occasionally to prevent sticking to the bottom of the pan.

5. Once cooked, remove from heat and let it sit, covered, for a few minutes.

6. Fluff the quinoa porridge with a fork and divide it into serving bowls.

7. Top with sliced bananas, berries, chopped nuts, coconut flakes, or any other desired toppings.

8. Serve warm and enjoy your wholesome breakfast quinoa porridge!

Nutritional info: (per serving, without toppings)

- Calories: 250

- Fat: 5g

- Carbohydrates: 45g

- Protein: 7g

- Fiber: 5g

Green Smoothie

Preparation time: 5 minutes

Cooking time: 0 minutes

Number of servings: 2

Ingredients:

- 2 cups spinach or kale (fresh or frozen)

- 1 ripe banana

- 1 cup chopped mango or pineapple (fresh or frozen)

- 1/2 avocado

- 1 cup almond milk (or any plant-based milk)

- 1 tablespoon chia seeds or ground flaxseeds

- Optional: a few ice cubes for extra chill

Directions:

1. Place all ingredients in a blender.

2. Blend until smooth and creamy, adding more liquid if needed to reach your desired consistency.

3. Taste and adjust sweetness or thickness by adding more fruit or liquid if necessary.

4. Pour into glasses and serve immediately.

Nutritional info: (per serving)

- Calories: 250

- Fat: 11g

- Carbohydrates: 35g

- Protein: 5g

- Fiber: 10g

Coconut Yogurt Parfait

Preparation time: 5 minutes

Cooking time: 0 minutes

Number of servings: 2

Ingredients:

- 2 cups dairy-free coconut yogurt

- 1 cup mixed berries (strawberries, blueberries, raspberries)

- 1/4 cup granola

- 2 tablespoons shredded coconut

- Optional: drizzle of honey or maple syrup

Directions:

1. In serving glasses or bowls, layer the coconut yogurt, mixed berries, and granola.

2. Repeat the layers until the glasses are filled.

3. Top with shredded coconut and a drizzle of honey or maple syrup if desired.

4. Serve immediately and enjoy your refreshing coconut yogurt parfait!

Nutritional info: (per serving)

- Calories: 250

- Fat: 10g

- Carbohydrates: 30g

- Protein: 6g

- Fiber: 5g

Tempeh Bacon with Toast

Preparation time: 10 minutes

Cooking time: 10 minutes

Number of servings: 2

Ingredients:

- 1 package (8 oz) tempeh, sliced thinly

- 2 tablespoons soy sauce or tamari

- 1 tablespoon maple syrup

- 1 tablespoon apple cider vinegar

- 1 teaspoon smoked paprika

- 1/2 teaspoon garlic powder

- 1 tablespoon olive oil

- 4 slices whole grain bread, toasted

Directions:

1. In a shallow dish, whisk together soy sauce or tamari, maple syrup, apple cider vinegar, smoked paprika, and garlic powder to make the marinade.

2. Dip the tempeh slices into the marinade, ensuring they are coated evenly.

3. Heat olive oil in a skillet over medium heat.

4. Place the marinated tempeh slices in the skillet and cook for about 3-4 minutes on each side until they are crispy and browned.

5. Remove from the skillet and drain excess oil on a paper towel.

6. Serve the tempeh bacon hot alongside toasted whole grain bread.

Nutritional info: (per serving, without bread)

- Calories: 220

- Fat: 12g

- Carbohydrates: 8g

- Protein: 20g

- Fiber: 5g

Vegan Breakfast Sausages

Preparation time: 15 minutes

Cooking time: 15 minutes

Number of servings: 4

Ingredients:

- 1 1/2 cups cooked brown lentils (drained if using canned)

- 1/2 cup breadcrumbs

- 1/4 cup finely chopped onion

- 2 cloves garlic, minced

- 2 tablespoons tomato paste

- 1 tablespoon soy sauce or tamari

- 1 teaspoon smoked paprika

- 1 teaspoon ground cumin

- 1/2 teaspoon dried thyme

- Salt and pepper to taste

- 2 tablespoons olive oil (for cooking)

Directions:

1. Preheat the oven to 375°F (190°C).

2. In a food processor, pulse the cooked lentils until they form a coarse paste.

3. Transfer the lentils to a mixing bowl and add breadcrumbs, finely chopped onion, minced garlic, tomato paste, soy sauce or tamari, smoked paprika, ground cumin, dried thyme, salt, and pepper. Mix until well combined.

4. Divide the mixture into portions and shape them into sausage-like patties.

5. Heat olive oil in a skillet over medium heat.

6. Cook the patties for about 3-4 minutes on each side until they are browned and cooked through.

7. Alternatively, you can bake the patties on a lightly greased baking sheet for 15-20 minutes, flipping halfway through.

8. Serve the vegan breakfast sausages hot alongside hash browns or your favorite breakfast sides.

Nutritional info: (per serving)

- Calories: 180

- Fat: 6g

- Carbohydrates: 24g

- Protein: 9g

- Fiber: 7g

Hash Browns

Preparation time: 15 minutes

Cooking time: 20 minutes

Number of servings: 4

Ingredients:

- 3 large russet potatoes, peeled and grated

- 1 small onion, finely chopped

- 2 tablespoons olive oil

- Salt and pepper to taste

- Optional: paprika or garlic powder for extra flavor

Directions:

1. Grate the peeled potatoes using a box grater or a food processor.

2. Place the grated potatoes in a clean kitchen towel and squeeze out as much excess moisture as possible.

3. In a mixing bowl, combine the grated potatoes with finely chopped onion, salt, and pepper. You can also add paprika or garlic powder for extra flavor if desired.

4. Heat olive oil in a skillet over medium heat.

5. Add a portion of the potato mixture to the skillet, shaping it into a round patty about 1/2 inch thick.

6. Cook for about 5-7 minutes on each side, or until golden brown and crispy.

7. Repeat the process with the remaining potato mixture.

8. Once cooked, transfer the hash browns to a plate lined with paper towels to drain any excess oil.

9. Serve the hash browns hot alongside the vegan breakfast sausages or as a standalone breakfast item.

Nutritional info: (per serving)

- Calories: 180

- Fat: 6g

- Carbohydrates: 30g

- Protein: 4g

- Fiber: 3g

Chapter 3

Lunch

Lentil Soup

Preparation time: 10 minutes

Cooking time: 40 minutes

Number of servings: 6

Ingredients:

- 1 cup dried green or brown lentils, rinsed

- 1 tablespoon olive oil

- 1 onion, finely chopped

- 2 carrots, diced

- 2 stalks celery, diced

- 3 cloves garlic, minced

- 1 teaspoon ground cumin

- 1 teaspoon ground coriander

- 6 cups vegetable or chicken broth

- Salt and pepper to taste

- Fresh chopped parsley for garnish (optional)

Directions:

1. Heat olive oil in a large pot over medium heat. Add chopped onion, carrots, and celery. Cook, stirring occasionally, until vegetables soften (about 5-7 minutes).

2. Add minced garlic, ground cumin, and ground coriander. Cook for an additional 1-2 minutes until fragrant.

3. Pour in the broth and add the rinsed lentils. Bring to a boil.

4. Reduce heat to a simmer, cover partially, and cook for about 30-35 minutes or until the lentils are tender.

5. Season with salt and pepper to taste.

6. Ladle into bowls, garnish with fresh parsley if desired, and serve hot.

   Nutritional info: (Per serving)

- Calories: 210

- Total Fat: 4.5g

- Saturated Fat: 0.5g

- Cholesterol: 0mg

- Sodium: 780mg

- Total Carbohydrate: 31g

- Dietary Fiber: 14g

- Total Sugars: 4g

- Protein: 12g

Quinoa Salad with Veggies

Preparation time: 20 minutes

Cooking time: 15 minutes (for quinoa)

Number of servings: 6

Ingredients:

- 1 cup quinoa, rinsed

- 2 cups water or vegetable broth

- 1 cucumber, diced

- 1 red bell pepper, diced

- 1 cup cherry tomatoes, halved

- 1/4 cup red onion, finely chopped

- 1/4 cup fresh parsley, chopped

- 1/4 cup olive oil

- 2 tablespoons lemon juice

- 2 cloves garlic, minced

- Salt and pepper to taste

- Optional: Feta cheese or crumbled goat cheese (for topping)

Directions:

1. In a saucepan, bring the water or vegetable broth to a boil. Add quinoa, reduce heat to low, cover, and simmer for 15 minutes or until liquid is absorbed and quinoa is cooked. Remove from heat and let it cool.

2. In a large bowl, combine the cooked and cooled quinoa, diced cucumber, red bell pepper, cherry tomatoes, red onion, and fresh parsley.

3. In a small bowl, whisk together olive oil, lemon juice, minced garlic, salt, and pepper to make the dressing.

4. Pour the dressing over the quinoa and vegetables. Toss gently to coat everything evenly.

5. Top with crumbled feta cheese or goat cheese if desired.

6. Serve immediately or refrigerate before serving.

Nutritional info: (Per serving, without optional toppings)

- Calories: 260

- Total Fat: 14g

- Saturated Fat: 2g

- Cholesterol: 0mg

- Sodium: 15mg

- Total Carbohydrate: 30g

- Dietary Fiber: 4g

- Total Sugars: 3g

- Protein: 6g

Vegan Buddha Bowl

Preparation time: 20 minutes

Cooking time: 30 minutes

Number of servings: 4

Ingredients:

- 1 cup quinoa, rinsed

- 2 cups water or vegetable broth

- 1 can (15 oz) chickpeas, drained and rinsed

- 2 tablespoons olive oil

- 1 teaspoon smoked paprika

- 1 teaspoon ground cumin

- Salt and pepper to taste

- 2 cups mixed greens (spinach, kale, or lettuce)

- 1 avocado, sliced

- 1 cup cherry tomatoes, halved

- 1 cucumber, sliced

- 1/4 cup hummus or tahini sauce

- Lemon wedges for serving (optional)

Directions:

1. In a saucepan, bring water or vegetable broth to a boil. Add quinoa, reduce heat to low, cover, and simmer for 15 minutes or until liquid is absorbed and quinoa is cooked. Set aside.

2. Preheat oven to 400°F (200°C).

3. Toss chickpeas with olive oil, smoked paprika, cumin, salt, and pepper. Spread them on a baking sheet and roast for 20-25 minutes or until crispy, shaking the pan occasionally.

4. Assemble the bowls by dividing the cooked quinoa, roasted chickpeas, mixed greens, avocado slices, cherry tomatoes, and cucumber among 4 bowls.

5. Drizzle each bowl with hummus or tahini sauce.

6. Serve with lemon wedges if desired.

Nutritional info: (Per serving)

- Calories: 480

- Total Fat: 20g

- Saturated Fat: 3g

- Cholesterol: 0mg

- Sodium: 380mg

- Total Carbohydrate: 62g

- Dietary Fiber: 16g

- Total Sugars: 6g

- Protein: 16g

Black Bean Tacos

Preparation time: 15 minutes

Cooking time: 15 minutes

Number of servings: 4

Ingredients:

1. 1 can (15 oz) black beans, drained and rinsed

2. 1 tablespoon olive oil

3. 1 onion, diced

4. 2 cloves garlic, minced

5. 1 teaspoon chili powder

6. 1/2 teaspoon ground cumin

7. Salt and pepper to taste

8. 8 small tortillas (corn or flour)

9. Toppings: shredded lettuce, diced tomatoes, sliced avocado, salsa, chopped cilantro, lime wedges

Directions:

1. Heat olive oil in a skillet over medium heat. Add diced onion and sauté until translucent.

2. Add minced garlic, chili powder, ground cumin, salt, and pepper. Cook for another minute until fragrant.

3. Stir in the black beans and cook for 5-7 minutes, mashing some of the beans with the back of a spoon or a fork.

4. Warm the tortillas in a dry skillet or microwave.

5. Fill each tortilla with the black bean mixture.

6. Top with shredded lettuce, diced tomatoes, sliced avocado, salsa, chopped cilantro, and serve with lime wedges.

Nutritional info: (Per serving, without toppings)

- Calories: 290

- Total Fat: 7g

- Saturated Fat: 1g

- Cholesterol: 0mg

- Sodium: 370mg

- Total Carbohydrate: 47g

- Dietary Fiber: 10g

- Total Sugars: 2g

- Protein: 11g

Vegetable Stir-Fry

Preparation time: 15 minutes

Cooking time: 15 minutes

Number of servings: 4

Ingredients:

- 2 tablespoons sesame oil

- 3 cups mixed vegetables (bell peppers, broccoli, carrots, snap peas, mushrooms, etc.), sliced or diced

- 3 cloves garlic, minced

- 1-inch piece of ginger, minced

- 1/4 cup low-sodium soy sauce or tamari

- 2 tablespoons rice vinegar

- 1 tablespoon honey or maple syrup (optional for sweetness)

- Cooked rice or quinoa for serving

Directions:

1. Heat sesame oil in a large skillet or wok over medium-high heat.

2. Add minced garlic and ginger, sauté for 30 seconds until fragrant.

3. Add the mixed vegetables and stir-fry for 5-7 minutes until they begin to soften but are still crisp.

4. In a small bowl, mix together soy sauce, rice vinegar, and honey or maple syrup (if using). Pour this sauce over the vegetables and toss to coat evenly.

5. Continue cooking for another 2-3 minutes until the sauce thickens slightly and coats the vegetables.

6. Serve the vegetable stir-fry over cooked rice or quinoa.

Nutritional info: (Per serving, without rice or quinoa)

- Calories: 120

- Total Fat: 7g

- Saturated Fat: 1g

- Cholesterol: 0mg

- Sodium: 720mg

- Total Carbohydrate: 12g

- Dietary Fiber: 4g

- Total Sugars: 6g

- Protein: 4g

Sweet Potato and Black Bean Chili

Preparation time: 15 minutes

Cooking time: 40 minutes

Number of servings: 6

Ingredients:

- 2 tablespoons olive oil

- 1 onion, chopped

- 3 cloves garlic, minced

- 2 medium sweet potatoes, peeled and diced

- 1 red bell pepper, diced

- 1 can (15 oz) black beans, drained and rinsed

- 1 can (14 oz) diced tomatoes

- 2 cups vegetable broth

- 2 teaspoons chili powder

- 1 teaspoon ground cumin

- 1 teaspoon paprika

- Salt and pepper to taste

Optional toppings: chopped cilantro, diced avocado, shredded cheese, sour cream or yogurt

Directions:

1. Heat olive oil in a large pot over medium heat. Add chopped onion and cook until translucent.

2. Add minced garlic and cook for another minute until fragrant.

3. Stir in diced sweet potatoes and red bell pepper, cook for 5 minutes.

4. Add black beans, diced tomatoes, vegetable broth, chili powder, ground cumin, paprika, salt, and pepper. Bring to a boil.

5. Reduce heat to low, cover, and simmer for 25-30 minutes or until sweet potatoes are tender.

6. Adjust seasoning if needed. Serve hot, garnished with chopped cilantro, diced avocado, shredded cheese, or a dollop of sour cream or yogurt if desired.

Nutritional info: (Per serving)

- Calories: 240

- Total Fat: 6g

- Saturated Fat: 1g

- Cholesterol: 0mg

- Sodium: 560mg

- Total Carbohydrate: 40g

- Dietary Fiber: 10g

- Total Sugars: 9g

- Protein: 8g

Mediterranean Hummus Wrap

Preparation time: 10 minutes

Cooking time: N/A

Number of servings: 2

Ingredients:

- 2 large whole wheat or spinach tortillas

- 1/2 cup hummus

- 1 cup mixed salad greens

- 1/2 cup diced cucumber

- 1/2 cup diced tomatoes

- 1/4 cup sliced red onion

- 1/4 cup sliced Kalamata olives

- 2 tablespoons crumbled feta cheese (optional)

- 2 tablespoons chopped fresh parsley or basil

- Olive oil and balsamic vinegar for drizzling (optional)

Directions:

1. Lay the tortillas flat on a clean surface.

2. Spread 1/4 cup of hummus onto each tortilla, leaving a border around the edges.

3. Layer mixed salad greens, diced cucumber, tomatoes, red onion, Kalamata olives, feta cheese (if using), and fresh herbs on top of the hummus.

4. Drizzle with olive oil and balsamic vinegar if desired.

5. Roll the tortillas tightly, tucking in the sides as you go.

6. Slice the wraps in half diagonally and serve.

Nutritional info: (Per serving)

- Calories: 350

- Total Fat: 14g

- Saturated Fat: 2g

- Cholesterol: 5mg

- Sodium: 760mg

- Total Carbohydrate: 45g

- Dietary Fiber: 10g

- Total Sugars: 5g

- Protein: 13g

Falafel with Tahini Sauce

Preparation time: 20 minutes

Cooking time: 15 minutes

Number of servings: Makes about 20 falafel

Ingredients:

For Falafel:

1. 2 cups cooked or canned chickpeas, drained and rinsed

2. 1/2 cup chopped fresh parsley

3. 1/2 cup chopped fresh cilantro

4. 1 small onion, chopped

5. 3 cloves garlic, minced

6. 1 teaspoon ground cumin

7. 1 teaspoon ground coriander

8. 1/2 teaspoon baking powder

9. 3 tablespoons all-purpose flour or chickpea flour

10. Salt and pepper to taste

11. Vegetable oil for frying

For Tahini Sauce:

- 1/4 cup tahini

- 2 tablespoons lemon juice

- 2 tablespoons water

- 1 clove garlic, minced

- Salt to taste

Directions:

For Falafel:

1. In a food processor, combine chickpeas, parsley, cilantro, chopped onion, minced garlic, cumin, coriander, baking

powder, flour, salt, and pepper. Pulse until the mixture is well combined but not pureed. It should have a coarse texture.

2. Shape the mixture into small balls or patties using your hands.

3. Heat vegetable oil in a frying pan over medium-high heat.

4. Fry the falafel in batches for about 3-4 minutes on each side until golden brown. Remove and drain on paper towels.

For Tahini Sauce:

1. In a small bowl, whisk together tahini, lemon juice, water, minced garlic, and salt until smooth. Adjust consistency by adding more water if needed.

2. Serve the falafel with the tahini sauce for dipping or inside pita bread with fresh vegetables and sauce.

Nutritional info: (Per 3 falafel, without sauce)

- Calories: 180

- Total Fat: 8g

- Saturated Fat: 1g

- Cholesterol: 0mg

- Sodium: 280mg

- Total Carbohydrate: 22g

- Dietary Fiber: 6g

- Total Sugars: 3g

- Protein: 7g

Stuffed Bell Peppers

Preparation time: 20 minutes

Cooking time: 50 minutes

Number of servings: 4

Ingredients:

- 4 large bell peppers, tops removed, seeds and membranes removed

- 1 tablespoon olive oil

- 1 onion, diced

- 2 cloves garlic, minced

- 1 cup cooked quinoa or rice

- 1 can (15 oz) black beans, drained and rinsed

- 1 can (14 oz) diced tomatoes

- 1 teaspoon chili powder

- 1 teaspoon cumin

- Salt and pepper to taste

- 1 cup shredded cheese (cheddar, mozzarella, or vegan cheese)

- Chopped fresh cilantro or parsley for garnish

Directions:

1. Preheat oven to 375°F (190°C).

2. Heat olive oil in a skillet over medium heat. Add diced onion and cook until translucent.

3. Add minced garlic, cooked quinoa or rice, black beans, diced tomatoes, chili powder, cumin, salt, and pepper. Stir and cook for 5-7 minutes until heated through.

4. Place the hollowed-out bell peppers in a baking dish. Spoon the quinoa and black bean mixture into the peppers.

5. Cover the dish with foil and bake for 30-35 minutes or until the peppers are tender.

6. Remove the foil, sprinkle shredded cheese on top of each pepper, and bake for an additional 5-10 minutes until the cheese is melted and bubbly.

7. Garnish with chopped cilantro or parsley before serving.

Nutritional info: (Per serving)

- Calories: 380

- Total Fat: 14g

- Saturated Fat: 6g

- Cholesterol: 30mg

- Sodium: 550mg

- Total Carbohydrate: 47g

- Dietary Fiber: 12g

- Total Sugars: 8g

- Protein: 18g

Spinach and Mushroom Pasta

Preparation time: 15 minutes

Cooking time: 20 minutes

Number of servings: 4

Ingredients:

- 8 oz pasta (spaghetti, fettuccine, or penne)

- 2 tablespoons olive oil

- 3 cloves garlic, minced

- 8 oz mushrooms, sliced

- 4 cups fresh spinach leaves

- 1/4 teaspoon red pepper flakes (optional)

- Salt and pepper to taste

- Grated Parmesan cheese or nutritional yeast for serving (optional)

Directions:

1. Cook the pasta according to package instructions. Drain and set aside.

2. In a large skillet, heat olive oil over medium heat. Add minced garlic and sauté for 30 seconds.

3. Add sliced mushrooms and cook for 5-7 minutes until they release their moisture and start to brown.

4. Stir in fresh spinach leaves and red pepper flakes (if using). Cook until the spinach wilts, about 2-3 minutes.

5. Add the cooked pasta to the skillet with the mushroom and spinach mixture. Toss to combine and heat through.

6. Season with salt and pepper to taste.

7. Serve hot, garnished with grated Parmesan cheese or nutritional yeast if desired.

Nutritional info: (Per serving)

- Calories: 320

- Total Fat: 9g

- Saturated Fat: 1g

- Cholesterol: 0mg

- Sodium: 25mg

- Total Carbohydrate: 51g

- Dietary Fiber: 5g

- Total Sugars: 3g

- Protein: 10g

Veggie Sushi Rolls

Preparation time: 30 minutes

Cooking time: N/A

Number of servings: Makes 4 rolls

Ingredients:

- 4 sheets nori seaweed

- 2 cups sushi rice, prepared according to package instructions

- 1 cucumber, julienned

- 1 avocado, thinly sliced

- 1 carrot, julienned

- 1 bell pepper (any color), thinly sliced

- 4-5 spears asparagus, blanched

- Soy sauce, pickled ginger, wasabi for serving

Directions:

1. Lay a sheet of nori on a bamboo sushi mat or a clean kitchen towel.

2. Spread a thin layer of prepared sushi rice over the nori, leaving a small border at the top edge.

3. Arrange cucumber, avocado slices, julienned carrot, bell pepper slices, and blanched asparagus near the bottom edge of the nori.

4. Start rolling the sushi tightly, using the bamboo mat or towel to help. Apply gentle pressure as you roll.

5. Seal the edge of the nori by moistening it slightly with water.

6. Repeat the process with the remaining nori sheets and ingredients.

7. Slice the rolls into bite-sized pieces using a sharp knife dipped
   in water.

8. Serve with soy sauce, pickled ginger, and wasabi.

   Nutritional info: (Per roll, without condiments)

- Calories: 220

- Total Fat: 5g

- Saturated Fat: 1g

- Cholesterol: 0mg

- Sodium: 120mg

- Total Carbohydrate: 40g

- Dietary Fiber: 7g

- Total Sugars: 3g

- Protein: 4g

Cauliflower Buffalo Wings

Preparation time: 20 minutes

Cooking time: 25 minutes

Number of servings: 4

Ingredients:

- 1 head cauliflower, cut into florets

- 3/4 cup all-purpose flour or chickpea flour (for gluten-free option)

- 3/4 cup unsweetened almond milk or other plant-based milk

- 1 teaspoon garlic powder

- 1 teaspoon onion powder

- 1/2 teaspoon smoked paprika

- Salt and pepper to taste

- 3/4 cup buffalo sauce (or your favorite hot sauce)

- 2 tablespoons melted vegan butter or olive oil

Directions:

1. Preheat the oven to 450°F (230°C). Line a baking sheet with parchment paper.

2. In a mixing bowl, whisk together flour, almond milk, garlic powder, onion powder, smoked paprika, salt, and pepper until you have a smooth batter.

3. Dip each cauliflower floret into the batter, ensuring it's evenly coated, and place it on the prepared baking sheet.

4. Bake for 20-25 minutes until the cauliflower is tender and the batter is slightly crispy.

5. In a separate bowl, mix buffalo sauce and melted vegan butter or olive oil.

6. Toss the baked cauliflower in the buffalo sauce mixture until evenly coated.

7. Return the coated cauliflower to the baking sheet and bake for an additional 5-7 minutes until crispy.

8. Serve hot with vegan ranch or blue cheese dressing and celery sticks.

Nutritional info: (Per serving)

- Calories: 180

- Total Fat: 7g

- Saturated Fat: 1g

- Cholesterol: 0mg

- Sodium: 1240mg

- Total Carbohydrate: 26g

- Dietary Fiber: 4g

- Total Sugars: 3g

- Protein: 4g

Vegan Pad Thai

Preparation time: 25 minutes

Cooking time: 15 minutes

Number of servings: 4

Ingredients:

- 8 oz rice noodles

- 2 tablespoons sesame oil

- 1 block (14 oz) firm tofu, pressed and cubed

- 2 cloves garlic, minced

- 1 red bell pepper, thinly sliced

- 1 cup shredded carrots

- 1 cup bean sprouts

- 3 green onions, chopped

- 1/4 cup roasted peanuts, chopped (optional, for garnish)

For the Sauce:

- 3 tablespoons soy sauce or tamari

- 2 tablespoons maple syrup or brown sugar

- 2 tablespoons lime juice

- 1 tablespoon rice vinegar

- 1 tablespoon Sriracha sauce (adjust to taste)

- 1 tablespoon peanut butter

- 1 teaspoon grated fresh ginger

- 2 cloves garlic, minced

Directions:

1. Cook rice noodles according to package instructions. Drain and set aside.

2. In a small bowl, whisk together all the sauce ingredients and set aside.

3. Heat sesame oil in a large skillet or wok over medium-high heat. Add cubed tofu and cook until golden brown on all sides. Remove from the skillet and set aside.

4. In the same skillet, add minced garlic, sliced bell pepper, and shredded carrots. Stir-fry for 2-3 minutes.

5. Add cooked noodles, tofu, bean sprouts, and the prepared sauce to the skillet. Toss everything together until well combined and heated through.

6. Remove from heat and garnish with chopped green onions and peanuts (if using).

7. Serve hot and enjoy!

   Nutritional info: (Per serving)

- Calories: 430

- Total Fat: 14g

- Saturated Fat: 2g

- Cholesterol: 0mg

- Sodium: 800mg

- Total Carbohydrate: 66g

- Dietary Fiber: 5g

- Total Sugars: 11g

- Protein: 12g

Curried Chickpea Salad

Preparation time: 15 minutes

Cooking time: N/A

Number of servings: 4

Ingredients:

- 2 cans (15 oz each) chickpeas, drained and rinsed

- 1/4 cup vegan mayonnaise or Greek yogurt

- 2 tablespoons curry powder

- 1 tablespoon lemon juice

- 2 stalks celery, finely chopped

- 1/4 cup red onion, finely chopped

- 1/4 cup raisins or dried cranberries

- Salt and pepper to taste

- Chopped fresh cilantro for garnish (optional)

Directions:

1. In a large mixing bowl, mash about half of the chickpeas with a fork or potato masher.

2. Add vegan mayonnaise or Greek yogurt, curry powder, lemon juice, chopped celery, red onion, and raisins or dried cranberries to the bowl.

3. Stir until all ingredients are well combined. If needed, add more mayo or yogurt for desired creaminess.

4. Season with salt and pepper to taste.

5. Garnish with chopped fresh cilantro if desired.

6. Serve the curried chickpea salad on sandwiches, wraps, salads, or enjoy it on its own.

Nutritional info: (Per serving)

- Calories: 320

- Total Fat: 9g

- Saturated Fat: 1g

- Cholesterol: 0mg

- Sodium: 520mg

- Total Carbohydrate: 47g

- Dietary Fiber: 12g

- Total Sugars: 10g

- Protein: 13g

Tomato Basil Soup with Grilled Cheese (Vegan)

Preparation time: 15 minutes

Cooking time: 25 minutes

Number of servings: 4

Ingredients:

For Tomato Basil Soup:

- 1 tablespoon olive oil

- 1 onion, chopped

- 3 cloves garlic, minced

- 2 cans (28 oz each) crushed tomatoes

- 2 cups vegetable broth

- 1/4 cup chopped fresh basil leaves

- Salt and pepper to taste

- 1/2 teaspoon red pepper flakes (optional)

For Vegan Grilled Cheese:

- 8 slices whole grain bread

- 1 cup vegan cheddar or mozzarella cheese, shredded

- Vegan butter or margarine

Directions:

For Tomato Basil Soup:

1. Heat olive oil in a pot over medium heat. Add chopped onion and sauté until translucent.

2. Add minced garlic and cook for another minute until fragrant.

3. Pour in the crushed tomatoes and vegetable broth. Bring to a simmer.

4. Add chopped basil leaves, salt, pepper, and red pepper flakes (if using). Simmer for 15-20 minutes.

5. Blend the soup using an immersion blender or transfer to a regular blender in batches to puree until smooth. Return to the pot and keep warm.

For Vegan Grilled Cheese:

1. Heat a skillet or griddle over medium heat.

2. Spread vegan butter on one side of each slice of bread.

3. Place one slice of bread, buttered side down, onto the skillet. Sprinkle a layer of vegan cheese on top and cover with another slice of bread, buttered side facing up.

4. Cook until the bottom slice is golden brown and the cheese starts melting. Flip the sandwich and cook until the other side is golden brown.

5. Repeat with the remaining slices of bread and cheese.

6. Serve the tomato basil soup hot with vegan grilled cheese sandwiches.

    Nutritional info: (Per serving of soup and 1 sandwich)

- Calories: 490

- Total Fat: 18g

- Saturated Fat: 4g

- Cholesterol: 0mg

- Sodium: 1250mg

- Total Carbohydrate: 68g

- Dietary Fiber: 13g

- Total Sugars: 18g

- Protein: 19g

Tofu Veggie Stir-Fry

Preparation time: 15 minutes

Cooking time: 15 minutes

Number of servings: 4

Ingredients:

- 1 block (14 oz) firm tofu, pressed and cubed

- 2 tablespoons sesame oil

- 3 cloves garlic, minced

- 1 inch ginger, grated

- 2 cups broccoli florets

- 1 bell pepper, thinly sliced

- 1 carrot, julienned

- 1 cup snap peas or snow peas

- 1/4 cup low-sodium soy sauce or tamari

- 2 tablespoons rice vinegar

- 1 tablespoon maple syrup or brown sugar

- 1 tablespoon cornstarch mixed with 2 tablespoons water (optional, for thickening)

- Cooked rice or quinoa for serving

Directions:

1. Heat sesame oil in a large skillet or wok over medium-high heat.

2. Add minced garlic and grated ginger. Sauté for 30 seconds.

3. Add cubed tofu to the skillet and cook until golden brown on all sides. Remove from the skillet and set aside.

4. In the same skillet, add broccoli florets, bell pepper slices, julienned carrot, and snap peas. Stir-fry for 3-4 minutes until the vegetables are tender-crisp.

5. In a small bowl, mix together soy sauce, rice vinegar, and maple syrup or brown sugar. Pour this sauce over the vegetables in the skillet.

6. If desired, add the cornstarch-water mixture to thicken the sauce. Cook for an additional minute.

7. Add the cooked tofu back to the skillet and toss everything together until well combined.

8. Serve the tofu veggie stir-fry over cooked rice or quinoa.

Nutritional info: (Per serving without rice or quinoa)

- Calories: 250

- Total Fat: 12g

- Saturated Fat: 2g

- Cholesterol: 0mg

- Sodium: 860mg

- Total Carbohydrate: 20g

- Dietary Fiber: 5g

- Total Sugars: 9g

- Protein: 18g

Avocado and White Bean Wrap

Preparation time: 15 minutes

Cooking time: N/A

Number of servings: 2

Ingredients:

- 1 ripe avocado, mashed
- 1 can (15 oz) white beans, drained and rinsed
- 2 tablespoons lemon juice
- 1/4 teaspoon garlic powder
- Salt and pepper to taste
- 2 large whole wheat or spinach tortillas
- 1 cup mixed salad greens
- 1/2 cucumber, sliced
- 1/2 cup shredded carrots
- 1/4 cup sliced red onion
- Optional: Sprouts, sunflower seeds, or chopped fresh herbs for added flavor

Directions:

1. In a bowl, combine mashed avocado, white beans, lemon juice, garlic powder, salt, and pepper. Mash some of the beans while leaving some whole for texture.

2. Lay the tortillas flat on a clean surface.

3. Spread the avocado and white bean mixture evenly over the tortillas, leaving a border around the edges.

4. Layer mixed salad greens, sliced cucumber, shredded carrots, red onion, and any additional toppings over the avocado and white bean mixture.

5. Roll the tortillas tightly, tucking in the sides as you go.

6. Slice the wraps in half diagonally and serve.

   Nutritional info: (Per serving)

- Calories: 380

- Total Fat: 12g

- Saturated Fat: 2g

- Cholesterol: 0mg

- Sodium: 620mg

- Total Carbohydrate: 58g

- Dietary Fiber: 17g

- Total Sugars: 4g

- Protein: 15g

Vegan Pesto Pasta

Preparation time: 15 minutes

Cooking time: 10 minutes

Number of servings: 4

Ingredients:

- 8 oz pasta of your choice (spaghetti, penne, etc.)

- 2 cups fresh basil leaves

- 1/3 cup pine nuts or walnuts

- 3 cloves garlic

- 1/4 cup nutritional yeast

- 1/4 cup olive oil

- 2 tablespoons lemon juice

- Salt and pepper to taste

- Cherry tomatoes and extra basil for garnish (optional)

Directions:

1. Cook the pasta according to package instructions. Drain and set aside, reserving some pasta water.

2. In a food processor, combine fresh basil, pine nuts or walnuts, garlic, nutritional yeast, olive oil, lemon juice, salt, and pepper. Pulse until a thick paste forms. If too thick, add a bit of reserved pasta water to loosen the pesto.

3. Toss the cooked pasta with the vegan pesto until well coated.

4. Garnish with halved cherry tomatoes and additional basil if desired.

5. Serve hot or at room temperature.

    Nutritional info: (Per serving)

- Calories: 420

- Total Fat: 20g

- Saturated Fat: 2g

- Cholesterol: 0mg

- Sodium: 10mg

- Total Carbohydrate: 52g

- Dietary Fiber: 4g

- Total Sugars: 2g

- Protein: 12g

Zucchini Noodles with Marinara Sauce

Preparation time: 15 minutes

Cooking time: 15 minutes

Number of servings: 2

Ingredients:

- 4 medium zucchinis, spiralized or cut into noodles

- 2 cups marinara sauce (store-bought or homemade)

- 1 tablespoon olive oil

- 2 cloves garlic, minced

- Salt and pepper to taste

- Fresh basil leaves for garnish (optional)

Directions:

1. Heat olive oil in a skillet over medium heat. Add minced garlic
   and sauté for 30 seconds until fragrant.

2. Add zucchini noodles to the skillet and toss gently for 2-3 minutes until just tender. Be careful not to overcook, as zucchini noodles can become mushy.

3. Pour marinara sauce over the zucchini noodles and toss until heated through.

4. Season with salt and pepper to taste.

5. Garnish with fresh basil leaves if desired.

6. Serve immediately.

   Nutritional info: (Per serving)

- Calories: 180

- Total Fat: 7g

- Saturated Fat: 1g

- Cholesterol: 0mg

- Sodium: 520mg

- Total Carbohydrate: 26g

- Dietary Fiber: 6g

- Total Sugars: 16g

- Protein: 5g

Veggie Burger with Sweet Potato Fries

Preparation time: 25 minutes

Cooking time: 40 minutes

Number of servings: 4

Ingredients:

For Veggie Burger:

- 2 cans (15 oz each) black beans, drained and rinsed

- 1 cup cooked quinoa

- 1/2 cup bread crumbs or oats

- 1/4 cup chopped red onion

- 2 cloves garlic, minced

- 2 tablespoons chopped fresh parsley

- 1 teaspoon ground cumin

- Salt and pepper to taste

- Burger buns and toppings of choice

For Sweet Potato Fries:

- 2 large sweet potatoes, peeled and cut into fries

- 2 tablespoons olive oil

- 1 teaspoon paprika

- 1/2 teaspoon garlic powder

- Salt and pepper to taste

Directions:

For Veggie Burger:

1. Preheat the oven to 375°F (190°C).

2. In a large bowl, mash half of the black beans with a fork or potato masher. Add the remaining black beans, cooked quinoa, bread crumbs or oats, red onion, minced garlic, chopped parsley, cumin, salt, and pepper. Mix until well combined.

3. Form the mixture into burger patties.

4. Heat a skillet over medium heat and cook the patties for 4-5 minutes on each side until golden brown.

For Sweet Potato Fries:

1. In a bowl, toss sweet potato fries with olive oil, paprika, garlic powder, salt, and pepper until coated.

2. Spread the fries on a baking sheet lined with parchment paper.

3. Bake for 20-25 minutes, flipping halfway through, until crispy.

4. Assemble the veggie burgers on buns with your favorite toppings and serve with sweet potato fries.

Nutritional info: (Per serving, without toppings)

Veggie Burger:

- Calories: 320

- Total Fat: 5g

- Saturated Fat: 1g

- Cholesterol: 0mg

- Sodium: 460mg

- Total Carbohydrate: 55g

- Dietary Fiber: 15g

- Total Sugars: 3g

- Protein: 17g

Sweet Potato Fries (per serving):

- Calories: 180

- Total Fat: 7g

- Saturated Fat: 1g

- Cholesterol: 0mg

- Sodium: 190mg

- Total Carbohydrate: 29g

- Dietary Fiber: 6g

- Total Sugars: 6g

- Protein: 3g

Portobello Mushroom Fajitas

Preparation time: 15 minutes

Cooking time: 15 minutes

Number of servings: 4

Ingredients:

- 4 large portobello mushrooms, stems removed, sliced

- 1 onion, sliced

- 1 red bell pepper, sliced

- 1 green bell pepper, sliced

- 2 cloves garlic, minced

- 2 tablespoons olive oil

- 2 teaspoons chili powder

- 1 teaspoon ground cumin

- 1 teaspoon smoked paprika

- Salt and pepper to taste

- 8 small flour or corn tortillas

- Optional toppings: Guacamole, salsa, chopped cilantro, lime wedges

Directions:

1. Heat olive oil in a skillet over medium-high heat.

2. Add sliced portobello mushrooms, onion, red bell pepper, green bell pepper, and minced garlic to the skillet. Sauté for 5-7 minutes until the vegetables are tender-crisp.

3. Sprinkle chili powder, ground cumin, smoked paprika, salt, and pepper over the veggies. Stir to coat evenly and cook for an additional 2-3 minutes.

4. Warm the tortillas in a separate skillet or oven.

5. Assemble the fajitas by spooning the mushroom and vegetable mixture onto the warmed tortillas.

6. Serve with optional toppings such as guacamole, salsa, chopped cilantro, and lime wedges.

Nutritional info: (Per serving, includes 2 fajitas)

- Calories: 280

- Total Fat: 9g

- Saturated Fat: 1g

- Cholesterol: 0mg

- Sodium: 310mg

- Total Carbohydrate: 45g

- Dietary Fiber: 7g

- Total Sugars: 6g

- Protein: 9g

Cucumber and Avocado Nori Rolls

Preparation time: 20 minutes

Cooking time: N/A

Number of servings: Makes 4 rolls

Ingredients:

- 4 nori seaweed sheets

- 2 cups sushi rice, prepared according to package instructions

- 1 ripe avocado, thinly sliced

- 1 cucumber, julienned

- 1/2 red bell pepper, thinly sliced

- 1/4 cup shredded carrots

- Soy sauce, wasabi, and pickled ginger for serving

Directions:

1. Lay a sheet of nori on a bamboo sushi mat or a clean kitchen towel.

2. Spread a thin layer of prepared sushi rice over the nori, leaving a small border at the top edge.

3. Arrange avocado slices, julienned cucumber, red bell pepper slices, and shredded carrots near the bottom edge of the nori.

4. Start rolling the sushi tightly, using the bamboo mat or towel to help. Apply gentle pressure as you roll.

5. Seal the edge of the nori by moistening it slightly with water.

6. Repeat the process with the remaining nori sheets and ingredients.

7. Slice the rolls into bite-sized pieces using a sharp knife dipped in water.

8. Serve with soy sauce, wasabi, and pickled ginger.

   Nutritional info: (Per roll, without condiments)

- Calories: 170

- Total Fat: 5g

- Saturated Fat: 1g

- Cholesterol: 0mg

- Sodium: 90mg

- Total Carbohydrate: 29g

- Dietary Fiber: 5g

- Total Sugars: 1g

- Protein: 4g

Vegan Pizza with Veggie Toppings

Preparation time: 20 minutes

Cooking time: 15 minutes

Number of servings: 4

Ingredients:

- 1 pre-made pizza crust or homemade vegan pizza dough

- 1/2 cup marinara sauce

- 1 cup vegan cheese (mozzarella or cheddar)

- 1 cup assorted veggies (sliced bell peppers, sliced onions, sliced mushrooms, cherry tomatoes, etc.)

- Fresh basil leaves for garnish (optional)

- Red pepper flakes (optional)

- Olive oil (for brushing the crust)

Directions:

1. Preheat the oven to 425°F (220°C).

2. Place the pizza crust on a baking sheet or pizza stone.

3. Spread marinara sauce evenly over the crust, leaving a small border around the edges.

4. Sprinkle vegan cheese over the sauce layer.

5. Top with assorted veggies of your choice.

6. Brush the edges of the crust with olive oil.

7. Bake in the preheated oven for 12-15 minutes until the crust is golden and the cheese is melted and bubbly.

8. Remove from the oven, garnish with fresh basil leaves and red pepper flakes if desired.

9. Slice and serve hot.

   Nutritional info: (Per serving, 1/4 of the pizza)

- Calories: 320

- Total Fat: 12g

- Saturated Fat: 2g

- Cholesterol: 0mg

- Sodium: 560mg

- Total Carbohydrate: 44g

- Dietary Fiber: 4g

- Total Sugars: 3g

- Protein: 9g

Eggplant and Chickpea Curry

Preparation time: 15 minutes

Cooking time: 30 minutes

Number of servings: 4

Ingredients:

- 2 tablespoons vegetable oil

- 1 onion, finely chopped

- 3 cloves garlic, minced

- 1 tablespoon fresh ginger, grated

- 1 eggplant, cut into cubes

- 1 can (15 oz) chickpeas, drained and rinsed

- 2 tomatoes, diced

- 1 teaspoon ground cumin

- 1 teaspoon ground coriander

- 1 teaspoon turmeric powder

- 1 teaspoon curry powder

- 1/2 teaspoon red chili powder (adjust to taste)

- 1 can (14 oz) coconut milk

- Salt to taste

- Fresh cilantro for garnish

Directions:

1. Heat vegetable oil in a large skillet or pot over medium heat.

2. Add chopped onion and sauté until translucent.

3. Add minced garlic and grated ginger. Sauté for another minute until fragrant.

4. Add cubed eggplant to the skillet and cook for 5-7 minutes until it starts to soften.

5. Stir in chickpeas, diced tomatoes, ground cumin, ground coriander, turmeric powder, curry powder, and red chili powder. Mix well to combine.

6. Pour in the coconut milk and bring the mixture to a simmer.

7. Reduce heat to low, cover the skillet, and let it simmer for 15-20 minutes until the eggplant is tender and the flavors have melded together.

8. Season with salt to taste.

9. Garnish with fresh cilantro before serving.

10. Serve the curry hot over rice or with naan bread.

Nutritional info: (Per serving)

Calories: 320

- Total Fat: 18g

- Saturated Fat: 12g

- Cholesterol: 0mg

- Sodium: 280mg

- Total Carbohydrate: 35g

- Dietary Fiber: 11g

- Total Sugars: 9g

- Protein: 8g

Chapter 4

Dinners

Quinoa Salad

Preparation time: 15 minutes

Cooking Time: 15 minutes

Number of servings: 4

Ingredients:

- 1 cup quinoa, rinsed

- 2 cups water or vegetable broth

- 1 red bell pepper, diced

- 1 cucumber, diced

- 1/4 cup red onion, finely chopped

- 1/4 cup fresh parsley, chopped

- 1/4 cup olive oil

- 2 tablespoons lemon juice

- 1 teaspoon ground cumin

- Salt and pepper to taste

- Optional: feta cheese or avocado for topping

Directions:

1. In a medium saucepan, bring water or vegetable broth to a boil. Add quinoa, reduce heat to low, cover, and simmer for 15 minutes or until liquid is absorbed and quinoa is fluffy.

2. In a large bowl, combine cooked quinoa, diced bell pepper, cucumber, red onion, and parsley.

3. In a small bowl, whisk together olive oil, lemon juice, ground cumin, salt, and pepper to make the dressing.

4. Pour the dressing over the quinoa mixture and toss to combine.

5. Top with crumbled feta cheese or sliced avocado if desired.

6. Serve chilled or at room temperature.

Nutritional Info:

- Calories: 290

- Total Fat: 14g

- Sodium: 20mg

- Total Carbohydrate: 35g

- Dietary Fiber: 5g

- Protein: 8g

Veggie Stir-Fry

Preparation time: 15 minutes

Cooking Time: 10 minutes

Number of servings: 4

Ingredients:

- 2 cups mixed vegetables (bell peppers, broccoli, carrots, snap peas, etc.), sliced

- 1 tablespoon sesame oil

- 3 cloves garlic, minced

- 1 tablespoon grated ginger

- 1/4 cup low-sodium soy sauce or tamari

- 2 tablespoons rice vinegar

- 1 tablespoon maple syrup or agave nectar

- 2 cups cooked brown rice or quinoa (for serving)

- Optional: sesame seeds for garnish

Directions:

1. Heat sesame oil in a large skillet or wok over medium-high heat.

2. Add minced garlic and grated ginger, stir for 30 seconds until fragrant.

3. Add sliced vegetables to the skillet and stir-fry for 3-5 minutes until they are tender-crisp.

4. In a small bowl, mix soy sauce, rice vinegar, and maple syrup. Pour the sauce over the vegetables and stir well to coat.

5. Continue cooking for another 2-3 minutes until the sauce thickens slightly.

6. Serve the stir-fry over cooked brown rice or quinoa. Sprinkle with sesame seeds if desired.

Nutritional Info:

- Calories: 180

- Total Fat: 4g

- Sodium: 480mg

- Total Carbohydrate: 32g

- Dietary Fiber: 5g

- Protein: 5g

Black Bean Tacos

Preparation time: 15 minutes

Cooking Time: 10 minutes

Number of servings: 4-6

Ingredients:

- 1 can (15 oz) black beans, drained and rinsed

- 1 tablespoon olive oil

- 1 onion, diced

- 2 cloves garlic, minced

- 1 teaspoon ground cumin

- 1 teaspoon chili powder

- Salt and pepper to taste

- Taco shells or tortillas

- Toppings: diced tomatoes, shredded lettuce, avocado, salsa, cilantro, lime wedges

Directions:

1. Heat olive oil in a skillet over medium heat. Add diced onion and minced garlic. Sauté until onion is translucent.

2. Add black beans, cumin, chili powder, salt, and pepper to the skillet. Cook for 5-7 minutes, stirring occasionally, until heated through.

3. Warm taco shells or tortillas according to package instructions.

4. Assemble tacos with the black bean mixture and desired toppings: diced tomatoes, shredded lettuce, avocado, salsa, cilantro, and a squeeze of lime juice.

Nutritional Info:

- Calories: 180
- Total Fat: 4g
- Sodium: 300mg
- Total Carbohydrate: 30g
- Dietary Fiber: 8g
- Protein: 8g

Sweet Potato Chili

Preparation time: 15 minutes

Cooking Time: 30 minutes

Number of servings: 6

Ingredients:

- 2 sweet potatoes, peeled and diced

- 1 onion, chopped

- 3 cloves garlic, minced

- 1 bell pepper, diced

- 1 can (15 oz) black beans, drained and rinsed

- 1 can (15 oz) kidney beans, drained and rinsed

- 1 can (14 oz) diced tomatoes

- 2 cups vegetable broth

- 2 tablespoons chili powder

- 1 teaspoon ground cumin

- 1 teaspoon paprika

- Salt and pepper to taste

- Optional toppings: diced avocado, chopped cilantro, vegan sour cream

Directions:

1. In a large pot or Dutch oven, sauté onion and garlic over medium heat until fragrant.

2. Add diced sweet potatoes, bell pepper, black beans, kidney beans, diced tomatoes, vegetable broth, chili powder, cumin, paprika, salt, and pepper.

3. Bring the mixture to a boil, then reduce heat to low and simmer for 25-30 minutes until sweet potatoes are tender.

4. Adjust seasoning to taste. Serve hot, garnished with diced avocado, chopped cilantro, and a dollop of vegan sour cream if desired.

Nutritional Info:

- Calories: 240

- Total Fat: 1g

- Sodium: 580mg

- Total Carbohydrate: 48g

- Dietary Fiber: 14g

- Protein: 12g

Cauliflower Wings

Preparation time: 15 minutes

Cooking Time: 25 minutes

Number of servings: 4

Ingredients:

- 1 head cauliflower, cut into florets

- 1 cup flour (all-purpose or chickpea flour for gluten-free option)

- 1 cup plant-based milk (such as almond or soy milk)

- 1 teaspoon garlic powder

- 1 teaspoon paprika

- 1/2 teaspoon cumin

- Salt and pepper to taste

- 1 cup bread crumbs (regular or panko for a crispier texture)

- BBQ sauce or hot sauce for coating

Directions:

1. Preheat the oven to 450°F (230°C). Line a baking sheet with parchment paper.

2. In a bowl, whisk together flour, plant-based milk, garlic powder, paprika, cumin, salt, and pepper to make a batter.

3. Dip each cauliflower floret into the batter, ensuring it's evenly coated, then roll it in bread crumbs to coat completely.

4. Place the coated florets on the prepared baking sheet. Bake for 20-25 minutes or until golden and crispy.

5. Once baked, toss the cauliflower wings in BBQ sauce or hot sauce of your choice until evenly coated.

6. Serve hot with your favorite dipping sauce.

Nutritional Info:

- Calories: 180

- Total Fat: 3g

- Sodium: 450mg

- Total Carbohydrate: 32g

- Dietary Fiber: 5g

- Protein: 7g

Spinach and Mushroom Risotto

Preparation time: 10 minutes

Cooking Time: 30 minutes

Number of servings: 4

Ingredients:

- 1 1/2 cups Arborio rice

- 4 cups vegetable broth

- 2 tablespoons olive oil

- 1 onion, finely chopped

- 2 cloves garlic, minced

- 8 oz mushrooms, sliced

- 4 cups fresh spinach leaves

- 1/2 cup nutritional yeast (optional, for a cheesy flavor)

- Salt and pepper to taste

- Fresh parsley for garnish

Directions:

1. In a saucepan, heat the vegetable broth and keep it warm on low heat.

2. In a large skillet or pot, heat olive oil over medium heat. Add chopped onion and minced garlic, sauté until softened.

3. Add Arborio rice to the skillet and stir for 1-2 minutes until lightly toasted.

4. Add a ladleful of warm vegetable broth to the rice, stirring frequently until the liquid is absorbed.

5. Continue adding the broth, one ladleful at a time, stirring often and allowing the rice to absorb the liquid before adding more. This process takes about 20-25 minutes.

6. When the rice is almost cooked, stir in the sliced mushrooms and spinach leaves. Cook for an additional 3-5 minutes until the vegetables are tender.

7. Remove from heat. Stir in nutritional yeast (if using), salt, and pepper.

8. Serve hot, garnished with fresh parsley.

Nutritional Info:

- Calories: 320

- Total Fat: 7g

- Sodium: 800mg

- Total Carbohydrate: 58g

- Dietary Fiber: 5g

- Protein: 8g

Vegan Pad Thai

Preparation time: 20 minutes

Cooking Time: 15 minutes

Number of servings: 4

Ingredients:

- 8 oz rice noodles

- 2 tablespoons oil

- 1 block (14 oz) firm tofu, pressed and cubed

- 3 cloves garlic, minced

- 1 cup broccoli florets

- 1 carrot, julienned

- 1 bell pepper, sliced

- 1 cup bean sprouts

- 3 green onions, chopped

- 1/4 cup chopped peanuts (optional for garnish)

- Lime wedges for serving

- Pad Thai Sauce:

- 3 tablespoons soy sauce or tamari

- 2 tablespoons maple syrup or brown sugar

- 2 tablespoons rice vinegar

- 1 tablespoon tamarind paste (or substitute with extra vinegar)

- 1 teaspoon sriracha sauce (adjust to taste)

Directions:

1. Cook rice noodles according to package instructions. Drain and set aside.

2. In a small bowl, whisk together the ingredients for the Pad Thai sauce.

3. Heat oil in a large skillet or wok over medium-high heat. Add cubed tofu and cook until golden brown. Remove tofu from the skillet and set aside.

4. In the same skillet, add minced garlic, broccoli, carrot, and bell pepper. Stir-fry for 3-4 minutes until vegetables are tender-crisp.

5. Add cooked noodles, tofu, bean sprouts, and green onions to the skillet.

6. Pour the Pad Thai sauce over the ingredients in the skillet. Toss everything together until well combined and heated through.

7. Serve hot, garnished with chopped peanuts (if using) and lime wedges.

Nutritional Info:

- Calories: 420

- Total Fat: 15g

- Sodium: 800mg

- Total Carbohydrate: 60g

- Dietary Fiber: 6g

- Protein: 15g

Zucchini Noodles with Pesto

Preparation time: 15 minutes

Cooking Time: 10 minutes

Number of servings: 2-3

Ingredients:

- 3-4 zucchinis, spiralized into noodles

- 1 cup fresh basil leaves

- 1/4 cup pine nuts

- 2 cloves garlic

- 1/4 cup olive oil

- 1/4 cup nutritional yeast (optional, for a cheesy flavor)

- Salt and pepper to taste

- Cherry tomatoes for garnish (optional)

Directions:

1. In a food processor, combine basil leaves, pine nuts, garlic, olive oil, nutritional yeast (if using), salt, and pepper. Blend until smooth to make the pesto sauce.

2. In a large pan, heat a little olive oil over medium heat. Add zucchini noodles and sauté for 2-3 minutes until just tender.

3. Add the prepared pesto sauce to the zucchini noodles and toss until evenly coated.

4. Cook for an additional 2 minutes until the pesto is heated through.

5. Serve hot, garnished with cherry tomatoes if desired.

Nutritional Info:

- Calories: 250

- Total Fat: 23g

- Sodium: 10mg

- Total Carbohydrate: 9g

- Dietary Fiber: 3g

- Protein: 5g

Stuffed Bell Peppers

Preparation time: 20 minutes

Cooking Time: 40 minutes

Number of servings: 4

Ingredients:

- 4 large bell peppers (any color), halved and seeds removed

- 1 cup cooked quinoa

- 1 can (15 oz) black beans, drained and rinsed

- 1 cup corn kernels

- 1 cup diced tomatoes

- 1/2 cup diced onion

- 2 cloves garlic, minced

- 1 teaspoon chili powder

- 1 teaspoon cumin

- Salt and pepper to taste

- Optional toppings: avocado, cilantro, vegan cheese

Directions:

1. Preheat the oven to 375°F (190°C).

2. In a bowl, mix together cooked quinoa, black beans, corn kernels, diced tomatoes, onion, minced garlic, chili powder, cumin, salt, and pepper.

3. Stuff each bell pepper half with the quinoa and veggie mixture.

4. Place the stuffed peppers on a baking dish and cover with foil.

5. Bake for 30-35 minutes, then remove the foil and bake for an additional 5-10 minutes until peppers are tender.

6. Serve hot, garnished with toppings like avocado, cilantro, or vegan cheese if desired.

Nutritional Info:

- Calories: 280

- Total Fat: 2g

- Sodium: 480mg

- Total Carbohydrate: 55g

- Dietary Fiber: 14g

- Protein: 14g

Eggplant Parmesan

Preparation time: 30 minutes

Cooking Time: 30 minutes

Number of servings: 4-6

Ingredients:

- 2 medium eggplants, sliced into 1/2-inch rounds

- 1 cup breadcrumbs (regular or panko)

- 1/2 cup grated vegan parmesan cheese

- 2 cups marinara sauce

- 1 cup vegan mozzarella cheese, shredded

- 2 tablespoons olive oil

- Salt and pepper to taste

- Fresh basil for garnish

Directions:

1. Preheat the oven to 375°F (190°C). Grease a baking sheet with olive oil.

2. In a bowl, mix breadcrumbs, grated vegan parmesan cheese, salt, and pepper.

3. Dip each eggplant slice into the breadcrumb mixture, ensuring it's coated evenly. Place them on the prepared baking sheet.

4. Bake the breaded eggplant slices for 20-25 minutes until golden brown and crispy.

5. In a baking dish, spread a thin layer of marinara sauce. Place a layer of baked eggplant slices on top, followed by more marinara sauce and shredded vegan mozzarella cheese. Repeat the layers.

6. Bake in the oven for another 20-25 minutes until the cheese is melted and bubbly.

7. Garnish with fresh basil before serving.

Nutritional Info:

- Calories: 320

- Total Fat: 14g

- Sodium: 780mg

- Total Carbohydrate: 42g

- Dietary Fiber: 12g

- Protein: 10g

Vegan Sushi Rolls

Preparation time: 30 minutes

Cooking Time: 20 minutes (for rice)

Number of servings: Makes 4-6 rolls

Ingredients:

- 2 cups sushi rice

- 4-6 nori sheets (seaweed)

- Assorted fillings: sliced avocado, cucumber strips, carrot matchsticks, bell pepper strips, tofu strips, etc.

- Soy sauce and pickled ginger for serving

- Wasabi paste (optional)

Directions:

1. Cook sushi rice according to package instructions and let it cool to room temperature.

2. Place a nori sheet shiny side down on a bamboo sushi mat or a clean kitchen towel.

3. Spread a thin layer of sushi rice on the nori sheet, leaving about 1 inch of the nori sheet empty at the top.

4. Arrange the fillings in a line across the center of the rice.

5. Roll the nori sheet tightly using the sushi mat, applying gentle pressure as you roll to seal it.

6. Wet the top edge of the nori sheet with a little water to seal the roll.

7. Repeat the process with the remaining ingredients.

8. Use a sharp knife to slice each roll into bite-sized pieces.

9. Serve with soy sauce, pickled ginger, and wasabi paste.

Nutritional Info:

- Calories: Varies

- Total Fat: Varies

- Sodium: Varies

- Total Carbohydrate: Varies

- Dietary Fiber: Varies

- Protein: Varies

Portobello Mushroom Burgers

Preparation time: 15 minutes

Cooking Time: 15 minutes

Number of servings: 2

Ingredients:

- 2 large portobello mushroom caps

- 2 burger buns (whole grain or gluten-free)

- 1/4 cup balsamic vinegar

- 2 tablespoons olive oil

- 2 cloves garlic, minced

- Salt and pepper to taste

- Toppings: lettuce, tomato slices, avocado slices, vegan mayo

Directions:

1. Clean the portobello mushroom caps and remove the stems.

2. In a bowl, whisk together balsamic vinegar, olive oil, minced garlic, salt, and pepper to make a marinade.

3. Place the mushroom caps in the marinade, turning to coat them evenly. Let them marinate for about 10 minutes.

4. Preheat a grill or grill pan over medium-high heat. Grill the mushroom caps for 5-7 minutes on each side until they are tender and grill marks appear.

5. Toast the burger buns if desired.

6. Assemble the burgers by placing the grilled portobello mushroom on the bun and adding your choice of toppings like lettuce, tomato, avocado, and vegan mayo.

7. Serve hot.

Nutritional Info:

- Calories: 250

- Total Fat: 14g

- Sodium: 20mg

- Total Carbohydrate: 25g

- Dietary Fiber: 4g

- Protein: 8g

Coconut Curry Tofu

Preparation time: 15 minutes

Cooking Time: 20 minutes

Number of servings: 4

Ingredients:

- 1 block (14 oz) firm tofu, pressed and cubed

- 1 tablespoon coconut oil

- 1 onion, chopped

- 3 cloves garlic, minced

- 1 tablespoon grated ginger

- 1 can (14 oz) coconut milk

- 2 tablespoons red curry paste

- 1 tablespoon soy sauce or tamari

- 1 tablespoon maple syrup or coconut sugar

- Assorted vegetables (bell peppers, broccoli, carrots, etc.)

- Cooked rice for serving

Directions:

1. Heat coconut oil in a large skillet or wok over medium heat. Add chopped onion, minced garlic, and grated ginger. Sauté until the onion is soft.

2. Add cubed tofu to the skillet and cook until golden brown on all sides.

3. Stir in red curry paste and cook for 1-2 minutes to toast the spices.

4. Pour in the coconut milk, soy sauce, and maple syrup. Stir to combine and bring to a simmer.

5. Add assorted vegetables to the skillet and cook until they are tender-crisp.

6. Simmer the curry for 5-7 minutes until the sauce thickens slightly.

7. Serve the coconut curry tofu over cooked rice.

Nutritional Info:

- Calories: 280

- Total Fat: 22g

- Sodium: 400mg

- Total Carbohydrate: 12g

- Dietary Fiber: 2g

- Protein: 12g

Avocado Toast

Preparation time: 5 minutes

Cooking Time: 5 minutes

Number of servings: 2

Ingredients:

- 2 ripe avocados

- 4 slices whole-grain bread

- 1-2 tablespoons olive oil

- Salt and pepper to taste

- Optional toppings: red pepper flakes, sliced tomatoes, microgreens, sesame seeds

Directions:

1. Toast the bread slices until they reach your desired level of crispiness.

2. While the bread is toasting, slice the avocados and scoop the flesh into a bowl.

3. Mash the avocado with a fork until it reaches your preferred consistency. Add salt and pepper to taste.

4. Once the toast is ready, drizzle each slice with a bit of olive oil.

5. Spread the mashed avocado evenly on the toast.

6. Add optional toppings like red pepper flakes, sliced tomatoes, microgreens, or sesame seeds for extra flavor and texture.

7. Serve immediately.

Nutritional Info:

- Calories: 250

- Total Fat: 18g

- Sodium: 150mg

- Total Carbohydrate: 20g

- Dietary Fiber: 8g

- Protein: 5g

Ratatouille

Preparation time: 20 minutes

Cooking Time: 40 minutes

Number of servings: 4-6

Ingredients:

- 1 eggplant, diced

- 2 zucchinis, diced

- 1 yellow squash, diced

- 1 onion, diced

- 2 bell peppers (red and yellow), diced

- 4 cloves garlic, minced

- 3 tomatoes, diced

- 2 tablespoons tomato paste

- 2 tablespoons olive oil

- 1 teaspoon dried thyme

- 1 teaspoon dried oregano

- Salt and pepper to taste

- Fresh basil for garnish

Directions:

1. Preheat the oven to 375°F (190°C).

2. In a large skillet, heat olive oil over medium heat. Add diced onion and minced garlic. Sauté until softened.

3. Add diced eggplant, zucchinis, yellow squash, bell peppers, tomatoes, tomato paste, dried thyme, dried oregano, salt, and pepper to the skillet. Stir to combine.

4. Cook for 5-7 minutes until the vegetables start to soften.

5. Transfer the mixture to a baking dish. Arrange the vegetables evenly.

6. Cover the dish with foil and bake for 25-30 minutes until the vegetables are tender.

7. Garnish with fresh basil before serving.

Nutritional Info:

- Calories: 120

- Total Fat: 5g

- Sodium: 50mg

- Total Carbohydrate: 18g

- Dietary Fiber: 7g

- Protein: 3g

Veggie Pizza

Preparation time: 20 minutes

Cooking Time: 15 minutes

Number of servings: 4

Ingredients:

- 1 prepared pizza dough (store-bought or homemade)

- 1/2 cup tomato sauce or marinara sauce

- 1 cup shredded vegan cheese or regular cheese

- Assorted vegetables (bell peppers, onions, mushrooms, spinach, etc.), sliced

- Olive oil for drizzling

- Italian seasoning, dried basil, or oregano for seasoning

Directions:

1. Preheat the oven to the temperature recommended for the pizza dough.

2. Roll out the pizza dough on a baking sheet or pizza stone.

3. Spread tomato sauce evenly over the dough, leaving a small border for the crust.

4. Sprinkle shredded cheese over the sauce.

5. Arrange sliced vegetables on top of the cheese.

6. Drizzle a little olive oil over the vegetables and sprinkle with Italian seasoning, dried basil, or oregano for extra flavor.

7. Bake the pizza according to the dough instructions until the crust is golden brown and the cheese is bubbly.

8. Remove from the oven, slice, and serve hot.

Nutritional Info:

- Calories: Varies

- Total Fat: Varies

- Sodium: Varies

- Total Carbohydrate: Varies

- Dietary Fiber: Varies

- Protein: Varies

Butternut Squash Soup

Preparation time: 15 minutes

Cooking Time: 40 minutes

Number of servings: 4-6

Ingredients:

- 1 medium butternut squash, peeled, seeded, and diced

- 1 onion, chopped

- 2 cloves garlic, minced

- 2 carrots, peeled and chopped

- 4 cups vegetable broth

- 1 teaspoon ground cumin

- 1/2 teaspoon ground cinnamon

- 1/4 teaspoon nutmeg

- Salt and pepper to taste

- 2 tablespoons olive oil

- Optional garnish: roasted pumpkin seeds, fresh herbs, drizzle
of cream

Directions:

1. Heat olive oil in a large pot over medium heat. Add chopped
onion and minced garlic. Sauté until softened.

2. Add diced butternut squash and carrots to the pot. Cook for
5-7 minutes, stirring occasionally.

3. Pour in the vegetable broth. Add ground cumin, cinnamon,
nutmeg, salt, and pepper. Bring to a boil, then reduce heat to
simmer for 20-25 minutes until the vegetables are tender.

4. Use an immersion blender or transfer the soup in batches to
a blender and puree until smooth.

5. Adjust seasoning if needed. If the soup is too thick, add more broth or water to reach the desired consistency.

6. Serve hot, garnished with roasted pumpkin seeds, fresh herbs, or a drizzle of cream if desired.

Nutritional Info:

- Calories: 150

- Total Fat: 5g

- Sodium: 550mg

- Total Carbohydrate: 27g

- Dietary Fiber: 6g

- Protein: 2g

Falafel Wraps

Preparation time: 20 minutes (plus time for soaking chickpeas)

Cooking Time: 15 minutes

Number of servings: Makes about 12 falafel

Ingredients:

- 1 cup dried chickpeas, soaked overnight
- 1 small onion, chopped
- 3 cloves garlic, minced
- 1/4 cup fresh parsley, chopped
- 1/4 cup fresh cilantro, chopped
- 1 teaspoon ground cumin
- 1 teaspoon ground coriander
- 1/2 teaspoon baking powder
- Salt and pepper to taste

- Oil for frying

- Pita bread or wraps

- Toppings: lettuce, tomatoes, cucumbers, tahini sauce

Directions:

1. Drain and rinse the soaked chickpeas. Pat them dry using a clean towel or paper towels.

2. In a food processor, combine chickpeas, chopped onion, minced garlic, parsley, cilantro, cumin, coriander, baking powder, salt, and pepper. Pulse until the mixture is coarse and well-combined.

3. Shape the mixture into small balls or patties.

4. Heat oil in a skillet over medium heat. Fry the falafel until they are golden brown and crispy on both sides (about 3-4 minutes per side).

5. Drain falafel on paper towels to remove excess oil.

6. Warm pita bread or wraps. Place falafel inside and add toppings like lettuce, tomatoes, cucumbers, and drizzle with tahini sauce.

7. Wrap tightly and serve immediately.

Nutritional Info:

- Calories: Varies

- Total Fat: Varies

- Sodium: Varies

- Total Carbohydrate: Varies

- Dietary Fiber: Varies

- Protein: Varies

Veggie Spring Rolls

Preparation time: 30 minutes

Cooking Time: None (requires assembly)

Number of servings: Makes about 8 spring rolls

Ingredients:

- 8 spring roll wrappers

- 2 cups thinly sliced vegetables (carrots, cucumber, bell peppers, lettuce, avocado, etc.)

- 1 cup cooked vermicelli noodles (optional)

- Fresh herbs (mint, cilantro, basil)

- Dipping sauce: soy sauce, peanut sauce, sweet chili sauce

Directions:

1. Prepare all the sliced vegetables, cooked vermicelli noodles, and fresh herbs.

2. Fill a large shallow bowl with warm water. Dip one spring roll wrapper into the water for a few seconds until it softens.

3. Lay the softened wrapper flat on a clean surface. Arrange a small amount of each filling ingredient in the center of the wrapper, leaving space on the sides.

4. Fold the sides of the wrapper over the filling, then roll it up tightly.

5. Repeat the process with the remaining wrappers and filling ingredients.

6. Serve the spring rolls with your choice of dipping sauce.

Nutritional Info:

- Calories: Varies

- Total Fat: Varies

- Sodium: Varies

- Total Carbohydrate: Varies

- Dietary Fiber: Varies

- Protein: Varies

Black Bean Burgers

Preparation time: 20 minutes

Cooking Time: 10 minutes

Number of servings: Makes 4 patties

Ingredients:

- 1 can (15 oz) black beans, drained and rinsed

- 1/2 cup bread crumbs

- 1/4 cup finely chopped onion

- 1/4 cup chopped bell peppers (any color)

- 2 cloves garlic, minced

- 1 teaspoon cumin

- 1 teaspoon paprika

- Salt and pepper to taste

- Olive oil for cooking

- Burger buns and toppings of your choice (lettuce, tomato, avocado, etc.)

Directions:

1. In a bowl, mash the black beans with a fork or potato masher until mostly smooth but still a bit chunky.

2. Add bread crumbs, chopped onion, chopped bell peppers, minced garlic, cumin, paprika, salt, and pepper to the mashed black beans. Mix until well combined.

3. Divide the mixture into 4 equal parts and shape each portion into a patty.

4. Heat a little olive oil in a skillet over medium heat. Cook the black bean patties for 4-5 minutes on each side until they are crispy and heated through.

5. Toast the burger buns if desired. Assemble the burgers with your favorite toppings.

6. Serve hot.

Nutritional Info:

- Calories: 200

- Total Fat: 3g

- Sodium: 350mg

- Total Carbohydrate: 35g

- Dietary Fiber: 9g

- Protein: 10g

Vegan Mac and Cheese

Preparation time: 15 minutes

Cooking Time: 15 minutes

Number of servings: 4

Ingredients:

- 2 cups elbow macaroni (or pasta of choice)

- 1 cup raw cashews, soaked in hot water for 1 hour

- 1 cup unsweetened almond milk (or any plant-based milk)

- 1/4 cup nutritional yeast

- 2 tablespoons lemon juice

- 2 tablespoons tahini

- 1 teaspoon garlic powder

- 1/2 teaspoon onion powder

- Salt and pepper to taste

- Optional: chopped fresh parsley for garnish

Directions:

1. Cook the macaroni according to package instructions. Drain
    and set aside.

2. In a blender, combine soaked cashews (drained), almond milk,
    nutritional yeast, lemon juice, tahini, garlic powder, onion
    powder, salt, and pepper. Blend until smooth and creamy.

3. Pour the cashew cheese sauce over the cooked macaroni. Stir
    to combine and coat the pasta evenly.

4. Heat the mac and cheese over low heat for a few minutes to
    warm it up if needed.

5. Serve hot, garnished with chopped fresh parsley if desired.

Nutritional Info:

- Calories: 400

- Total Fat: 17g

- Sodium: 100mg

- Total Carbohydrate: 48g

- Dietary Fiber: 4g

- Protein: 15g

Rainbow Buddha Bowl

Preparation time: 20 minutes

Cooking Time: 20 minutes (for grains, if using)

Number of servings: 2-3

Ingredients:

- Cooked grains (quinoa, rice, or couscous)

- 1 cup cooked chickpeas

- 1 cup roasted sweet potatoes, diced

- 1 cup steamed broccoli florets

- 1 cup shredded purple cabbage

- 1 large carrot, julienned or grated

- 1 avocado, sliced

- 2 tablespoons hummus or tahini dressing

- Sesame seeds for garnish

Directions:

1. Prepare grains according to package instructions if not already cooked.

2. Assemble bowls with cooked grains as the base.

3. Arrange cooked chickpeas, roasted sweet potatoes, steamed broccoli, shredded purple cabbage, julienned carrots, and sliced avocado in sections over the grains.

4. Drizzle hummus or tahini dressing over the bowls.

5. Sprinkle sesame seeds on top for garnish.

6. Serve immediately.

Nutritional Info:

- Calories: Varies

- Total Fat: Varies

- Sodium: Varies

- Total Carbohydrate: Varies

- Dietary Fiber: Varies

- Protein: Varies

Kale Caesar Salad

Preparation time: 15 minutes

Cooking Time: None

Number of servings: 4

Ingredients:

- 1 bunch kale, stems removed and leaves chopped

- 1 cup croutons (store-bought or homemade)

- 1/4 cup vegan Caesar dressing

- 1/4 cup nutritional yeast (optional, for added flavor)

- 1/4 cup sliced cherry tomatoes

- 2 tablespoons capers (optional)

- Lemon wedges for garnish

Directions:

1. In a large mixing bowl, add chopped kale leaves.

2. Pour vegan Caesar dressing over the kale. Massage the dressing into the kale leaves for a few minutes to soften them.

3. Add croutons, nutritional yeast (if using), sliced cherry tomatoes, and capers to the bowl.

4. Toss everything together until well combined.

5. Divide into individual servings and garnish with lemon wedges.

6. Serve immediately.

Nutritional Info:

- Calories: 180

- Total Fat: 5g

- Sodium: 350mg

- Total Carbohydrate: 25g

- Dietary Fiber: 4g

Chapter 5

Appetizers

Fruit Salad

Preparation time: 15 minutes

Number of servings: 4

Ingredients:

- 2 apples, diced

- 2 bananas, sliced

- 1 cup strawberries, sliced

- 1 cup grapes, halved

- 1 cup blueberries

- Juice of 1 lemon

- 2 tablespoons maple syrup or honey (optional)

Directions:

1. In a large bowl, combine all the prepared fruits.

2. Squeeze the lemon juice over the fruits and drizzle with maple syrup or honey if desired.

3. Gently toss the fruits until they're evenly coated.

4. Refrigerate for at least 30 minutes before serving.

Nutritional Info (per serving):

- Calories: 120

- Total Fat: 0.5g

- Carbohydrates: 30g

- Protein: 1g

Nut Butter Energy Balls

Preparation time: 15 minutes

Number of servings: 12 balls

Ingredients:

- 1 cup rolled oats

- 1/2 cup nut butter (almond, peanut, or cashew)

- 1/4 cup maple syrup or agave nectar

- 1/4 cup ground flaxseed

- 1 teaspoon vanilla extract

- 1/4 cup mini dairy-free chocolate chips or chopped nuts (optional)

Directions:

1. In a mixing bowl, combine all the ingredients until thoroughly mixed.

2. If the mixture is too dry, add a bit more nut butter or maple syrup. If too wet, add more oats.

3. Take about a tablespoon of the mixture and roll it into balls using your hands.

4. Place the balls on a plate or baking sheet lined with parchment paper.

5. Refrigerate for at least 30 minutes before serving.

Nutritional Info (per ball):

- Calories: 120

- Total Fat: 6g

- Carbohydrates: 12g

- Protein: 3g

Guacamole with Whole Grain Tortilla Chips

Preparation time: 10 minutes

Number of servings: 4

Ingredients:

- 3 ripe avocados

- 1 tomato, diced

- 1/2 onion, finely chopped

- 1/4 cup cilantro, chopped

- Juice of 1 lime

- Salt and pepper to taste

- Whole grain tortilla chips for serving

Directions:

1. Cut the avocados in half, remove the pits, and scoop the flesh
   into a bowl.

2. Mash the avocados with a fork until smooth or to your desired consistency.

3. Add diced tomato, chopped onion, cilantro, lime juice, salt, and pepper. Mix well.

4. Taste and adjust seasoning if needed.

5. Serve the guacamole with whole grain tortilla chips.

Nutritional Info (per serving, without chips):

- Calories: 160

- Total Fat: 14g

- Carbohydrates: 10g

- Protein: 2g

Chia Seed Pudding

Preparation time: 5 minutes (plus chilling time)

Number of servings: 2

Ingredients:

- 1/4 cup chia seeds

- 1 cup unsweetened almond milk (or any plant-based milk)

- 1-2 tablespoons maple syrup or agave syrup

- 1/2 teaspoon vanilla extract

- Fresh fruits or nuts for topping (optional)

Directions:

1. In a bowl or jar, mix together chia seeds, almond milk, maple syrup, and vanilla extract.

2. Stir well to combine and ensure there are no clumps of chia seeds.

3. Cover the bowl or jar and refrigerate for at least 2-3 hours, or preferably overnight.

4. Stir the mixture again before serving. If it's too thick, you can add a bit more almond milk to reach your desired consistency.

5. Top with fresh fruits or nuts if desired before serving.

Nutritional Info (per serving):

- Calories: 150

- Total Fat: 8g

- Carbohydrates: 15g

- Protein: 5g

Vegan Cheese and Crackers

Preparation time: 10 minutes

Number of servings: Varies

Ingredients:

- Vegan cheese of your choice (store-bought or homemade)

- Whole grain crackers or rice crackers

Directions:

1. Arrange the vegan cheese on a platter.

2. Place the whole grain crackers or rice crackers alongside the cheese.

3. Serve immediately.

Nutritional Info (varies based on cheese and crackers used):

- This can vary significantly based on the types and brands of vegan cheese and crackers used.

Edamame Beans

Preparation time: 10 minutes

Cooking Time: 5 minutes

Number of servings: 4

Ingredients:

- 2 cups frozen edamame beans (in pods)

- 1 tablespoon sesame oil

- Sea salt (optional)

Directions:

1. Boil the edamame beans in salted water for about 5 minutes or until tender. Drain and set aside.

2. Heat sesame oil in a pan over medium heat.

3. Add the cooked edamame beans to the pan and sauté for 2-3 minutes, stirring occasionally.

4. Sprinkle with a bit of sea salt if desired.

5. Remove from heat and serve warm.

Nutritional Info (per serving):

- Calories: 100

- Total Fat: 4g

- Carbohydrates: 8g

- Protein: 8g

Kale Chips

Preparation time: 10 minutes

Cooking Time: 15-20 minutes

Number of servings: 4

Ingredients:

- 1 bunch kale, washed and dried

- 1-2 tablespoons olive oil

- Salt and pepper to taste

- Optional: nutritional yeast, garlic powder, or other seasonings

Directions:

1. Preheat your oven to 300°F (150°C).

2. Remove the tough stems from the kale leaves and tear the leaves into bite-sized pieces.

3. In a large bowl, toss the kale with olive oil, making sure each piece is lightly coated.

4. Sprinkle with salt, pepper, and any other desired seasonings.

5. Spread the kale in a single layer on a baking sheet lined with parchment paper.

6. Bake for 15-20 minutes or until the edges are browned and crispy but not burnt.

7. Let them cool for a few minutes before serving.

Nutritional Info (per serving):

- Calories: 50

- Total Fat: 3g

- Carbohydrates: 5g

- Protein: 2g

Coconut Yogurt Parfait

Preparation time: 10 minutes

Number of servings: 2

Ingredients:

1 cup coconut yogurt

1/2 cup granola (check for a plant-based option)

1 cup mixed berries (strawberries, blueberries, raspberries)

Directions:

1. In serving glasses or bowls, layer the coconut yogurt, granola, and mixed berries.

2. Repeat the layers until the glasses are filled or until all ingredients are used.

3. Serve immediately or refrigerate until ready to eat.

Nutritional Info (per serving):

- Calories: 250

- Total Fat: 10g

- Carbohydrates: 35g

- Protein: 5g

Sliced Apples with Almond Butter

Preparation time: 5 minutes

Number of servings: 2

Ingredients:

- 2 apples, cored and sliced

- 4 tablespoons almond butter (or any nut/seed butter of choice)

- Optional toppings: cinnamon, chia seeds, or shredded coconut

Directions:

1. Arrange the apple slices on a plate.

2. Serve alongside almond butter for dipping or spreading on the slices.

3. Optionally, sprinkle with cinnamon, chia seeds, or shredded coconut.

Nutritional Info (per serving):

- Calories: 250

- Total Fat: 16g

- Carbohydrates: 25g

- Protein: 5g

Quinoa Salad Cups

Preparation time: 20 minutes

Cooking Time: 15 minutes

Number of servings: 6

Ingredients:

- 1 cup quinoa, rinsed

- 2 cups vegetable broth or water

- 1 cucumber, diced

- 1 bell pepper, diced

- 1 cup cherry tomatoes, halved

- 1/4 cup red onion, finely chopped

- 1/4 cup fresh parsley, chopped

- Juice of 1 lemon

- 3 tablespoons olive oil

- Salt and pepper to taste

- Lettuce leaves or endive leaves for cups

Directions:

1. In a medium saucepan, combine quinoa and vegetable broth/water. Bring to a boil, then reduce heat, cover, and simmer for 15 minutes or until quinoa is cooked and liquid is absorbed. Let it cool.

2. In a large bowl, mix together the cooked quinoa, cucumber, bell pepper, cherry tomatoes, red onion, and parsley.

3. In a small bowl, whisk together lemon juice, olive oil, salt, and pepper. Pour this dressing over the quinoa salad and toss to combine.

4. Spoon the quinoa salad into lettuce leaves or endive leaves to create cups.

5. Serve immediately or refrigerate until ready to serve.

Nutritional Info (per serving):

- Calories: 220

- Total Fat: 8g

- Carbohydrates: 30g

- Protein: 6g

Popcorn with Nutritional Yeast

Preparation time: 10 minutes

Cooking Time: 5 minutes

Number of servings: 4

Ingredients:

1/2 cup popcorn kernels

2 tablespoons coconut oil or olive oil

3 tablespoons nutritional yeast

Salt to taste

Directions:

1. Heat the coconut oil in a large pot over medium-high heat.

2. Add the popcorn kernels, cover with a lid, and shake the pot occasionally while the popcorn pops.

3. Once the popping slows down, remove the pot from the heat.

4. Transfer the popcorn to a large bowl.

5. Drizzle the popcorn with a bit more melted coconut oil or olive oil if desired.

6. Sprinkle with nutritional yeast and salt, tossing to coat evenly.

7. Serve immediately.

Nutritional Info (per serving):

- Calories: 120

- Total Fat: 7g

- Carbohydrates: 11g

- Protein: 4g

Rice Cakes with Mashed Banana and Cinnamon

Preparation time: 5 minutes

Number of servings: 2

Ingredients:

- 2 rice cakes

- 1 ripe banana

- 1/2 teaspoon ground cinnamon

Directions:

1. In a bowl, mash the ripe banana with a fork until smooth.

2. Spread the mashed banana evenly onto each rice cake.

3. Sprinkle ground cinnamon over the banana layer.

4. Serve immediately.

Nutritional Info (per serving):

- Calories: 110

- Total Fat: 0.5g

- Carbohydrates: 26g

- Protein: 2g

Stuffed Bell Peppers with Quinoa and Veggies

Preparation time: 15 minutes

Cooking Time: 30 minutes

Number of servings: 4

Ingredients:

- 4 bell peppers, any color, tops removed and seeded

- 1 cup cooked quinoa

- 1 cup mixed vegetables (such as diced zucchini, carrots, corn, peas)

- 1 can (15 oz) black beans, drained and rinsed

- 1 cup tomato sauce or marinara sauce

- 1 teaspoon cumin

- 1 teaspoon paprika

- Salt and pepper to taste

- Vegan cheese (optional)

Directions:

1. Preheat your oven to 375°F (190°C).

2. In a large bowl, mix together cooked quinoa, mixed vegetables, black beans, tomato sauce, cumin, paprika, salt, and pepper.

3. Stuff each bell pepper with the quinoa and veggie mixture.

4. Place the stuffed peppers in a baking dish. If using vegan cheese, sprinkle it on top of each stuffed pepper.

5. Cover the baking dish with foil and bake for 25-30 minutes or until the peppers are tender.

6. Remove the foil and bake for an additional 5 minutes to lightly brown the tops.

7. Serve hot.

Nutritional Info (per serving):

- Calories: 250

- Total Fat: 2g

- Carbohydrates: 50g

- Protein: 10g

Vegan Trail Mix (nuts, seeds, dried fruits)

Preparation time: 5 minutes

Number of servings: Varies

Ingredients:

- 1 cup mixed nuts (almonds, cashews, walnuts)

- 1/2 cup pumpkin seeds

- 1/2 cup sunflower seeds

- 1/2 cup dried cranberries or raisins

- 1/4 cup dried apricots, chopped

Directions:

1. In a bowl, mix together all the ingredients.

2. Adjust the proportions of nuts, seeds, and dried fruits to your preference.

3. Store the trail mix in an airtight container for snacking.

Nutritional Info (per serving):

- This can vary significantly based on the specific ingredients and proportions used.

Sweet Potato Fries

Preparation time: 15 minutes

Cooking Time: 25 minutes

Number of servings: 4

Ingredients:

- 2 large sweet potatoes, peeled and cut into fries

- 2 tablespoons olive oil

- 1 teaspoon paprika

- 1/2 teaspoon garlic powder

- Salt and pepper to taste

Directions:

1. Preheat your oven to 425°F (220°C) and line a baking sheet with parchment paper.

2. In a large bowl, toss the sweet potato fries with olive oil, paprika, garlic powder, salt, and pepper until evenly coated.

3. Spread the fries in a single layer on the prepared baking sheet.

4. Bake for 20-25 minutes, flipping the fries halfway through, until they are golden and crispy.

5. Remove from the oven and let them cool slightly before serving.

Nutritional Info (per serving):

- Calories: 180

- Total Fat: 7g

- Carbohydrates: 28g

- Protein: 2g

Vegan Sushi Rolls

Preparation time: 30 minutes

Cooking Time: Varies

Number of servings: Varies

Ingredients:

- 2 cups sushi rice, cooked and seasoned with rice vinegar, sugar, and salt

- Nori seaweed sheets

- Assorted vegetables (avocado, cucumber, carrot sticks, bell pepper strips, etc.)

- Extra fillings (tofu strips, marinated mushrooms, pickled radish, etc.)

- Soy sauce or tamari for dipping

- Wasabi and pickled ginger (optional)

Directions:

1. Lay a sheet of nori shiny side down on a bamboo sushi mat or a clean kitchen towel.

2. Spread a thin layer of sushi rice over the nori, leaving about 1-inch of the nori sheet uncovered at the top.

3. Arrange your choice of vegetables and fillings in a line across the center of the rice.

4. Using the bamboo mat or towel, tightly roll the nori sheet, applying gentle pressure to shape it into a roll.

5. Wet the uncovered edge of the nori sheet to seal the roll.

6. Repeat with the remaining ingredients.

7. Once the rolls are made, use a sharp knife to slice them into bite-sized pieces.

8. Serve with soy sauce, wasabi, and pickled ginger if desired.

Nutritional Info (varies based on ingredients and servings):

- Calories, fat, carbohydrates, and protein content can vary widely based on the specific ingredients used.

Zucchini Fritters

Preparation time: 15 minutes

Cooking Time: 15 minutes

Number of servings: 4

Ingredients:

- 2 medium zucchinis, grated
- 1/2 teaspoon salt
- 1/4 cup chickpea flour or all-purpose flour
- 2 tablespoons nutritional yeast
- 1/4 teaspoon garlic powder
- 1/4 teaspoon onion powder
- Black pepper to taste
- Olive oil for frying

Directions:

1. Place the grated zucchini in a colander, sprinkle with salt, and let it sit for about 10 minutes. Then squeeze out the excess moisture using a clean kitchen towel or paper towels.

2. In a mixing bowl, combine the grated zucchini, chickpea flour, nutritional yeast, garlic powder, onion powder, and black pepper. Mix well to form a batter.

3. Heat a thin layer of olive oil in a non-stick skillet over medium heat.

4. Scoop about 2 tablespoons of the zucchini batter and place it in the skillet, flattening it slightly with a spatula to form a fritter. Repeat for the remaining batter, leaving space between fritters in the skillet.

5. Cook the fritters for about 3-4 minutes on each side or until golden brown and crispy.

6. Remove the fritters from the skillet and place them on a plate lined with paper towels to absorb excess oil.

7. Serve the zucchini fritters warm.

Nutritional Info (per serving):

- Calories: 70

- Total Fat: 3g

- Carbohydrates: 8g

Chapter 6

Treats

Dairy-Free Cheesecake

Preparation time: 20 minutes

Chilling Time: 4-6 hours

Number of servings: 8-10

Ingredients:

For the Crust:

- 1 1/2 cups of crushed graham crackers (or vegan alternative)

- 1/4 cup of melted coconut oil

- 2 tablespoons of maple syrup or agave nectar

For the Filling:

- 2 cups of raw cashews (soaked in water for at least 4 hours, then drained)

- 1/2 cup of coconut cream

- 1/3 cup of maple syrup or agave nectar

- 1/4 cup of lemon juice

- 1 teaspoon of vanilla extract

- Pinch of salt

Directions:

Crust:

1. Preheat the oven to 350°F (175°C).

2. In a bowl, mix together the crushed graham crackers, melted coconut oil, and maple syrup.

3. Press the mixture into the bottom of a greased 9-inch springform pan.

4. Bake the crust for 10 minutes. Remove and let it cool.

Filling:

1. In a food processor or blender, blend the soaked cashews, coconut cream, maple syrup, lemon juice, vanilla extract, and salt until smooth and creamy.

2. Pour the filling over the cooled crust and smooth the top.

3. Place the cheesecake in the refrigerator and chill for at least 4-6 hours, or until set.

4. Once set, slice and serve. Optionally, top with fresh fruit or a fruit compote.

Nutritional Info:

- Calories: 402

- Total Fat: 27.6g

- Carbohydrates: 34.7g

- Fiber: 1.5g

- Protein: 7.3g

- Sugar: 17.5g

Coconut Milk Pudding

Preparation time: 5 minutes

Cooking Time: 10 minutes

Chilling Time: 2-3 hours

Number of servings: 4

Ingredients:

- 1 can (13.5 oz) coconut milk

- 3 tablespoons cornstarch

- 1/4 cup sugar or sweetener of choice

- 1 teaspoon vanilla extract

- Pinch of salt

- Optional toppings: toasted coconut flakes, fresh berries

Directions:

1. In a saucepan, whisk together the coconut milk, cornstarch, sugar, vanilla extract, and salt until smooth.

2. Place the saucepan over medium heat, stirring continuously until the mixture thickens, about 8-10 minutes.

3. Remove from heat and let it cool for a few minutes.

4. Pour the pudding into serving dishes or ramekins.

5. Cover and refrigerate for 2-3 hours until set.

6. Serve chilled, topped with toasted coconut flakes or fresh berries if desired.

Nutritional Info:

- Calories: 247

- Total Fat: 20g

- Carbohydrates: 15g

- Fiber: 0.4g

- Protein: 1.8g

- Sugar: 12g

Chia Seed Pudding

Preparation time: 5 minutes

Chilling Time: 2-4 hours or overnight

Number of servings: 2

Ingredients:

- 1/4 cup chia seeds

- 1 cup coconut milk (or any non-dairy milk)

- 1 tablespoon maple syrup or sweetener of choice

- 1/2 teaspoon vanilla extract

- Optional toppings: fresh fruit, nuts, or shredded coconut

Directions:

1. In a bowl, mix together the chia seeds, coconut milk, maple syrup, and vanilla extract.

2. Whisk the mixture thoroughly to avoid clumps.

3. Cover the bowl and refrigerate for at least 2-4 hours or overnight, allowing the chia seeds to absorb the liquid and form a pudding-like consistency.

4. Stir the pudding before serving and add your choice of toppings like fresh fruit, nuts, or shredded coconut.

Nutritional Info:

- Calories: 220

- Total Fat: 15g

- Carbohydrates: 18g

- Fiber: 11g

- Protein: 5g

- Sugar: 4g

Vegan Banana Bread

Preparation time: 15 minutes

Baking Time: 50-60 minutes

Number of servings: 8

Ingredients:

- 3 ripe bananas, mashed

- 1/3 cup melted coconut oil or vegetable oil

- 1/2 cup coconut sugar or brown sugar

- 1 teaspoon vanilla extract

- 1 1/2 cups all-purpose flour

- 1 teaspoon baking soda

- 1/2 teaspoon salt

- 1/2 teaspoon ground cinnamon (optional)

- 1/4 cup non-dairy milk (such as almond or soy)

Directions:

1. Preheat your oven to 350°F (175°C). Grease a 9x5-inch loaf pan.

2. In a mixing bowl, combine the mashed bananas, melted coconut oil, sugar, and vanilla extract.

3. Sift in the flour, baking soda, salt, and cinnamon (if using). Mix until just combined.

4. Add the non-dairy milk and mix until the batter is smooth.

5. Pour the batter into the prepared loaf pan.

6. Bake for 50-60 minutes or until a toothpick inserted into the center comes out clean.

7. Allow the banana bread to cool in the pan for 10-15 minutes before transferring it to a wire rack to cool completely.

Nutritional Info:

- Calories: 235

- Total Fat: 9g

- Carbohydrates: 37g

- Fiber: 2.5g

- Protein: 3g

- Sugar: 16g

Dairy-Free Brownies

Preparation time: 15 minutes

Baking Time: 20-25 minutes

Number of servings: 12

Ingredients:

- 1 cup all-purpose flour

- 1 cup coconut sugar or brown sugar

- 1/2 cup unsweetened cocoa powder

- 1/2 teaspoon baking powder

- 1/4 teaspoon salt

- 1/2 cup vegetable oil

- 1/4 cup unsweetened applesauce

- 1 teaspoon vanilla extract

- 1/4 cup dairy-free chocolate chips (optional)

Directions:

1. Preheat your oven to 350°F (175°C). Grease or line an 8x8-inch baking pan.

2. In a bowl, whisk together the flour, sugar, cocoa powder, baking powder, and salt.

3. Add the vegetable oil, applesauce, and vanilla extract to the dry ingredients. Mix until well combined.

4. Fold in the chocolate chips, if using.

5. Pour the batter into the prepared baking pan and spread it evenly.

6. Bake for 20-25 minutes or until a toothpick inserted into the center comes out with a few crumbs (not wet batter).

7. Let the brownies cool completely in the pan before cutting into squares.

Nutritional Info:

- Calories: 190

- Total Fat: 10g

- Carbohydrates: 25g

- Fiber: 2g

- Protein: 2g

- Sugar: 15g

Vegan Cupcakes

Preparation time: 15 minutes

Baking Time: 18-20 minutes

Number of servings: 12 cupcakes

Ingredients:

- 1 1/2 cups all-purpose flour

- 1 cup granulated sugar

- 1 teaspoon baking soda

- 1/2 teaspoon salt

- 1 cup almond milk (or any non-dairy milk)

- 1/3 cup vegetable oil

- 1 tablespoon apple cider vinegar or white vinegar

- 1 teaspoon vanilla extract

Directions:

1. Preheat your oven to 350°F (175°C). Line a muffin tin with cupcake liners.

2. In a mixing bowl, whisk together the flour, sugar, baking soda, and salt.

3. In a separate bowl, mix together the almond milk, vegetable oil, vinegar, and vanilla extract.

4. Pour the wet ingredients into the dry ingredients and mix until just combined. Do not overmix.

5. Divide the batter evenly among the cupcake liners, filling each about two-thirds full.

6. Bake for 18-20 minutes or until a toothpick inserted into the center of a cupcake comes out clean.

7. Allow the cupcakes to cool in the pan for a few minutes before transferring them to a wire rack to cool completely before frosting.

Nutritional Info:

- Calories: 180

- Total Fat: 6g

- Carbohydrates: 30g

- Fiber: 1g

- Protein: 2g

- Sugar: 16g

Dairy-Free Tiramisu

Preparation time: 30 minutes

Chilling Time: 4 hours or overnight

Number of servings: 8

Ingredients:

- 1 cup strong brewed coffee, cooled

- 2 tablespoons rum or coffee liqueur (optional)

- 1 package ladyfinger cookies (make sure they're vegan)

- 1 1/2 cups dairy-free cream cheese

- 1/2 cup powdered sugar

- 1 teaspoon vanilla extract

- Cocoa powder, for dusting

Directions:

1. In a shallow dish, combine the cooled coffee and rum or liqueur, if using.

2. Dip each ladyfinger cookie briefly into the coffee mixture and line the bottom of an 8x8-inch dish with a single layer of soaked cookies.

3. In a mixing bowl, beat the dairy-free cream cheese, powdered sugar, and vanilla extract until smooth and creamy.

4. Spread half of the cream cheese mixture over the layer of ladyfingers.

5. Repeat with another layer of soaked ladyfingers on top of the cream cheese layer, followed by the remaining cream cheese mixture.

6. Cover and refrigerate the tiramisu for at least 4 hours or overnight to allow the flavors to meld.

7. Before serving, dust the top with cocoa powder using a fine-mesh sieve.

Nutritional Info:

- Calories: 320

- Total Fat: 16g

- Carbohydrates: 40g

- Fiber: 1g

- Protein: 5g

- Sugar: 18g

Vegan Ice Cream (made with coconut milk or other non-dairy alternatives)

Preparation time: 10 minutes

Churning Time: 25-30 minutes

Freezing Time: 4-6 hours

Number of servings: 4

Ingredients:

- 1 can (13.5 oz) full-fat coconut milk or non-dairy milk of choice

- 1/2 cup sugar or sweetener of choice

- 1 teaspoon vanilla extract

- Optional add-ins: chopped nuts, dairy-free chocolate chips, fruit puree

Directions:

1. In a bowl, whisk together the coconut milk, sugar, and vanilla extract until the sugar is dissolved.

2. Pour the mixture into an ice cream maker and churn according to the manufacturer's instructions, usually 25-30 minutes until it reaches a soft-serve consistency.

3. If desired, add in any optional ingredients during the last few minutes of churning.

4. Transfer the churned ice cream into a freezer-safe container, smooth the top, and cover it with a lid or plastic wrap.

5. Freeze the ice cream for 4-6 hours or until firm.

6. Let the ice cream sit at room temperature for a few minutes before scooping and serving.

Nutritional Info:

- Calories: 240

- Total Fat: 17g

- Carbohydrates: 24g

- Fiber: 0g

- Protein: 1g

- Sugar: 24g

Dairy-Free Rice Pudding

Preparation time: 5 minutes

Cooking Time: 30 minutes

Number of servings: 4

Ingredients:

- 1/2 cup uncooked rice (short or long-grain)

- 3 cups non-dairy milk (coconut, almond, soy, etc.)

- 1/4 cup sugar or sweetener of choice

- 1 teaspoon vanilla extract

- 1/4 teaspoon ground cinnamon (optional)

- Pinch of salt

- Optional toppings: cinnamon powder, raisins, chopped nuts

Directions:

1. Rinse the rice under cold water until the water runs clear.

2. In a saucepan, combine the rice, non-dairy milk, sugar, vanilla extract, cinnamon (if using), and a pinch of salt.

3. Bring the mixture to a gentle boil over medium heat, then reduce the heat to low.

4. Simmer uncovered, stirring occasionally, for about 25-30 minutes or until the rice is tender and the mixture has thickened.

5. Remove from heat and let it sit for a few minutes to thicken further.

6. Serve warm or chilled, topped with cinnamon powder, raisins, or chopped nuts if desired.

Nutritional Info:

- Calories: 210

- Total Fat: 5g

- Carbohydrates: 36g

- Fiber: 1g

- Protein: 3g

- Sugar: 12g

Vegan Lemon Bars

Preparation time: 20 minutes

Baking Time: 40-45 minutes

Chilling Time: 2 hours

Number of servings: 12 bars

Ingredients:

For the Crust:

- 1 1/2 cups all-purpose flour

- 1/2 cup powdered sugar

- 1/2 cup melted coconut oil or vegan butter

For the Lemon Filling:

- 1 cup granulated sugar

- 1/4 cup cornstarch

- 1/2 cup lemon juice (about 3-4 lemons)

- Zest of 2 lemons

- 1/2 cup non-dairy milk (coconut, almond, soy, etc.)

- Powdered sugar for dusting (optional)

Directions:

1. Preheat your oven to 350°F (175°C). Grease or line an 8x8-inch baking pan.

2. In a bowl, mix together the flour, powdered sugar, and melted coconut oil or vegan butter until crumbly.

3. Press the mixture evenly into the bottom of the prepared baking pan.

4. Bake the crust for 15-18 minutes or until lightly golden. Remove from the oven and let it cool slightly.

5. In another bowl, whisk together the granulated sugar, cornstarch, lemon juice, lemon zest, and non-dairy milk until smooth.

6. Pour the lemon mixture over the baked crust.

7. Bake for an additional 25-30 minutes or until the edges are set and the center is slightly jiggly.

8. Remove from the oven and let it cool to room temperature, then refrigerate for at least 2 hours to set.

9. Once chilled, dust the top with powdered sugar if desired and cut into bars.

Nutritional Info:

- Calories: 220

- Total Fat: 9g

- Carbohydrates: 33g

- Fiber: 0.5g

- Protein: 1g

- Sugar: 19g

Dairy-Free Pumpkin Pie

Preparation time: 20 minutes

Baking Time: 55-60 minutes

Chilling Time: 4 hours or overnight

Number of servings: 8

Ingredients:

For the Crust:

- 1 1/4 cups graham cracker crumbs (use a vegan variety if needed)
- 1/4 cup melted coconut oil or vegan butter

For the Filling:

- 1 can (15 oz) pumpkin puree
- 1/2 cup full-fat coconut milk (from a can)
- 1/2 cup brown sugar or coconut sugar
- 1/4 cup cornstarch or arrowroot powder
- 1 teaspoon vanilla extract
- 1 teaspoon ground cinnamon
- 1/2 teaspoon ground ginger
- 1/4 teaspoon ground nutmeg

- 1/4 teaspoon ground cloves

- Pinch of salt

Directions:

Crust:

1. Preheat your oven to 350°F (175°C).

2. In a bowl, mix together the graham cracker crumbs and melted coconut oil or vegan butter until well combined.

3. Press the mixture into the bottom and sides of a 9-inch pie dish.

4. Bake the crust for 8-10 minutes. Remove from the oven and let it cool slightly.

Filling:

1. In a large mixing bowl, whisk together all the filling ingredients until smooth.

2. Pour the filling into the pre-baked crust.

3. Bake the pie in the preheated oven for 55-60 minutes or until the center is almost set.

4. Remove from the oven and let it cool completely on a wire rack.

5. Refrigerate the pie for at least 4 hours or overnight before serving.

Nutritional Info:

- Calories: 280

- Total Fat: 15g

- Carbohydrates: 34g

- Fiber: 2g

- Protein: 2g

- Sugar: 19g

Vegan Peanut Butter Cookies

Preparation time: 15 minutes

Baking Time: 10-12 minutes

Number of servings: 16 cookies

Ingredients:

- 1 cup peanut butter (creamy or crunchy)

- 3/4 cup granulated sugar

- 1 teaspoon vanilla extract

- 1 tablespoon non-dairy milk (if needed for consistency)

- Optional: pinch of salt, dairy-free chocolate chips or chopped nuts for topping

Directions:

1. Preheat your oven to 350°F (175°C). Line a baking sheet with parchment paper.

2. In a mixing bowl, combine the peanut butter, sugar, and vanilla extract. Mix until well combined. If the mixture seems too thick, add a tablespoon of non-dairy milk to achieve a smooth dough.

3. Roll the dough into small balls and place them on the prepared baking sheet, spacing them apart.

4. Use a fork to create a crisscross pattern on the cookies, gently pressing down on each ball to flatten it.

5. If desired, press chocolate chips or chopped nuts into the tops of the cookies.

6. Bake for 10-12 minutes or until the edges are slightly golden.

7. Let the cookies cool on the baking sheet for a few minutes before transferring them to a wire rack to cool completely.

Nutritional Info:

- Calories: 150

- Total Fat: 9g

- Carbohydrates: 15g

- Fiber: 1g

- Protein: 4g

- Sugar: 11g

Almond Flour Cake

Preparation time: 15 minutes

Baking Time: 30-35 minutes

Number of servings: 8

Ingredients:

- 2 cups almond flour

- 1/4 cup coconut flour

- 1 teaspoon baking powder

- 1/4 teaspoon salt

- 1/2 cup maple syrup or agave nectar

- 1/4 cup melted coconut oil or vegetable oil

- 4 flax eggs (4 tablespoons ground flaxseed + 10 tablespoons water, mixed and left to sit for 5 minutes)

- 1 teaspoon vanilla extract

- Optional: sliced almonds for topping

Directions:

1. Preheat your oven to 350°F (175°C). Grease or line an 8-inch round cake pan.

2. In a bowl, whisk together the almond flour, coconut flour, baking powder, and salt.

3. In another bowl, mix together the maple syrup, melted coconut oil, flax eggs, and vanilla extract.

4. Combine the wet and dry ingredients until well incorporated.

5. Pour the batter into the prepared cake pan and smooth the
    top.

6. Optionally, sprinkle sliced almonds on top of the batter.

7. Bake for 30-35 minutes or until a toothpick inserted into the
    center comes out clean.

8. Allow the cake to cool in the pan for 10-15 minutes before
    transferring it to a wire rack to cool completely.

Nutritional Info:

- Calories: 320

- Total Fat: 23g

- Carbohydrates: 25g

- Fiber: 4g

- Protein: 8g

- Sugar: 15g

Dairy-Free Chocolate Mousse

Preparation time: 15 minutes

Chilling Time: 2 hours

Number of servings: 4

Ingredients:

- 1 can (13.5 oz) full-fat coconut milk, chilled in the refrigerator overnight

- 1/4 cup cocoa powder

- 1/4 cup powdered sugar or sweetener of choice

- 1 teaspoon vanilla extract

- Vegan chocolate shavings or berries for garnish (optional)

Directions:

1. Open the can of chilled coconut milk without shaking it. Scoop out the solid coconut cream into a mixing bowl, leaving the liquid behind (save it for other recipes or smoothies).

2. Add cocoa powder, powdered sugar, and vanilla extract to the coconut cream.

3. Using a hand mixer or a stand mixer, whip the ingredients together until it forms stiff peaks and resembles a mousse-like texture.

4. Spoon the chocolate mousse into serving dishes or glasses.

5. Chill in the refrigerator for at least 2 hours before serving.

6. Garnish with vegan chocolate shavings or berries if desired before serving.

Nutritional Info:

- Calories: 240

- Total Fat: 19g

- Carbohydrates: 15g

- Fiber: 3g

- Protein: 3g

- Sugar: 9g

Vegan Apple Crisp

Preparation time: 15 minutes

Baking Time: 40-45 minutes

Number of servings: 6

Ingredients:

- 4-5 medium-sized apples, peeled, cored, and sliced

- 1 tablespoon lemon juice

- 1/4 cup maple syrup or agave nectar

- 1 teaspoon ground cinnamon

- 1/4 teaspoon ground nutmeg

- 1 cup rolled oats

- 1/2 cup almond flour

- 1/4 cup melted coconut oil or vegan butter

- 1/4 cup chopped nuts (optional)

Directions:

1. Preheat your oven to 350°F (175°C). Grease an 8x8-inch baking dish.

2. In a bowl, toss the sliced apples with lemon juice, maple syrup, cinnamon, and nutmeg until the apples are evenly coated. Transfer the mixture to the prepared baking dish.

3. In another bowl, combine the rolled oats, almond flour, melted coconut oil or vegan butter, and chopped nuts if using. Mix until crumbly.

4. Spread the oat mixture evenly over the apples in the baking dish.

5. Bake for 40-45 minutes or until the top is golden brown and the apples are tender.

6. Allow the apple crisp to cool for a few minutes before serving.

Nutritional Info:

- Calories: 240

- Total Fat: 12g

- Carbohydrates: 33g

- Fiber: 6g

- Protein: 3g

- Sugar: 18g

Dairy-Free Mango Sticky Rice

Preparation time: 10 minutes

Cooking Time: 20 minutes

Number of servings: 4

Ingredients:

- 1 cup glutinous rice (sticky rice), soaked for 1-2 hours and drained

- 1 can (13.5 oz) coconut milk

- 1/4 cup sugar

- Pinch of salt

- 2 ripe mangoes, peeled and sliced

- Toasted sesame seeds or shredded coconut for garnish (optional)

Directions:

1. In a saucepan, combine the soaked and drained glutinous rice with 1 1/4 cups of water. Bring it to a boil, then reduce the heat to low, cover, and let it simmer for 15-20 minutes or until the rice is tender and the water is absorbed.

2. In another saucepan, combine the coconut milk, sugar, and a pinch of salt. Heat the mixture over medium heat, stirring until the sugar is dissolved and the mixture is heated through but not boiling.

3. Remove the saucepan from the heat and pour half of the coconut milk mixture over the cooked sticky rice. Mix well to coat the rice thoroughly.

4. Let the rice sit for a few minutes to absorb the coconut milk.

5. To serve, spoon portions of the sweetened sticky rice onto plates or bowls, top with sliced mangoes, and drizzle with the remaining coconut milk mixture.

6. Garnish with toasted sesame seeds or shredded coconut if desired.

Nutritional Info:

- Calories: 350

- Total Fat: 18g

- Carbohydrates: 48g

- Fiber: 3g

- Protein: 3g

- Sugar: 22g

Vegan Oatmeal Cookies

Preparation time: 15 minutes

Baking Time: 10-12 minutes

Number of servings: 12 cookies

Ingredients:

- 1 cup rolled oats

- 3/4 cup whole wheat flour or all-purpose flour

- 1/2 teaspoon baking soda

- 1/2 teaspoon ground cinnamon

- 1/4 teaspoon salt

- 1/4 cup melted coconut oil or vegetable oil

- 1/4 cup maple syrup or agave nectar

- 1/4 cup unsweetened applesauce

- 1 teaspoon vanilla extract

- 1/2 cup dried fruits or nuts (optional)

Directions:

1. Preheat your oven to 350°F (175°C). Line a baking sheet with parchment paper.

2. In a bowl, mix together the rolled oats, flour, baking soda, cinnamon, and salt.

3. In another bowl, whisk together the melted coconut oil, maple syrup, applesauce, and vanilla extract until well combined.

4. Combine the wet and dry ingredients, stirring until a dough forms. If using, fold in dried fruits or nuts.

5. Scoop out portions of the dough and form them into balls. Place them on the prepared baking sheet and flatten them slightly with your hand or a fork.

6. Bake for 10-12 minutes or until the edges turn golden brown.

7. Let the cookies cool on the baking sheet for a few minutes before transferring them to a wire rack to cool completely.

Nutritional Info:

- Calories: 120

- Total Fat: 5g

- Carbohydrates: 18g

- Fiber: 1.5g

- Protein: 2g

- Sugar: 6g

Dairy-Free Berry Parfait

Preparation time: 10 minutes

Assembling Time: 5 minutes

Number of servings: 2

Ingredients:

- 1 cup dairy-free yogurt (coconut, almond, soy, etc.)

- 1 cup mixed fresh berries (strawberries, blueberries, raspberries)

- 1/4 cup granola (check for dairy-free options or make your own)

- 1 tablespoon maple syrup or agave nectar (optional)

Directions:

1. In two serving glasses or bowls, layer the dairy-free yogurt and mixed fresh berries alternately.

2. Drizzle a little maple syrup or agave nectar over the berries if you prefer extra sweetness.

3. Top the parfait with a layer of granola for added crunch.

4. Repeat the layers if your glasses allow or create multiple parfaits.

5. Serve immediately and enjoy!

Nutritional Info:

- Calories: 180

- Total Fat: 5g

- Carbohydrates: 30g

- Fiber: 4g

- Protein: 4g

Conclusion

Dear Reader,

As we come to the end of this culinary expedition through the vibrant world of plant-based eating, I hope these pages have not just been a guidebook but a catalyst for transformation in your kitchen and beyond.

Throughout this journey, we've ventured beyond the realm of mere recipes. We've explored the intricate dance of flavors and textures, the symphony of colors, and the nourishing embrace of ingredients gifted to us by the earth.

In the chapters preceding this conclusion, we embarked on a voyage of understanding the essence of a plant-based diet. We unveiled the science behind the food we consume, dismantling myths and misconceptions. We discovered the sheer variety and versatility of plant-based ingredients, each bite offering a tapestry of nutrients and vitality.

Breakfasts welcomed the dawn with zestful energy, infusing your mornings with healthful delights. Lunches became an opportunity to refuel your body, introducing an array of satisfying and invigorating meals. Dinners, oh the dinners! They transformed mundane evenings into feasts of culinary brilliance, proving that plant-based eating is a canvas for gastronomic artistry.

Beyond these main meals, we explored the realms of Appetizers that teased the palate and Treats that sweetened life's moments. From the first tantalizing bite to the last lingering taste, each dish celebrated the abundance and diversity that nature graciously offers.

But this journey wasn't solely about food; it was about empowerment. It was about realizing the immense impact our choices have—not just on our health but on the planet we call home. Choosing a plant-based lifestyle isn't merely a culinary preference; it's a commitment to sustainability, compassion, and holistic well-being.

As you close this book, remember that this isn't an endpoint but a threshold to endless possibilities. Let these recipes be your foundation, your starting point. Feel free to innovate, experiment, and make them your own. Let your kitchen be a playground where creativity dances with nutrition, and every meal becomes an expression of your values and tastes.

Beyond the recipes, let this journey guide you toward a deeper connection with the food you consume. Explore local produce, embrace seasonal flavors, and revel in the joy of mindful eating. Let each meal be an ode to gratitude—for the nourishment it provides and the positive impact it generates.

Thank you for entrusting me as your culinary companion. It's been an honor and a pleasure to share this adventure with you. May the flavors linger, the lessons enrich, and may your journey towards vibrant health and conscious living continue to blossom.

Wishing you abundance in every bite and fulfillment in every mindful meal.

With heartfelt gratitude and warmest wishes,

Francis A. Carter